STAYING
IN THE GAME

STAYING IN THE GAME

How to Keep Young and Active

RAY SIEGENER

HOUGHTON MIFFLIN COMPANY BOSTON 1980

For Dad ... approaching his 80th year ...
and still very much "in the game"

I wish to express my thanks to Jackie Aher for her assistance in preparing many of the illustrations for this book.

Library of Congress Cataloging in Publication Data
Siegener, Ray.
    Staying in the game.
    Bibliography: p.
    1. Aging. 2. Physical fitness. 3. Exercise
for aged. I. Title.
HQ106.S485   613.7   80-14776
ISBN 0-395-27596-2

Printed in the United States of America

S 10 9 8 7 6 5 4 3 2 1

Contents

2095072

Foreword

Old myths die hard. Most people still equate old age with disability. Ray Siegener's book *Staying in the Game* disproves this belief very effectively. The writer stresses that continued physical activity can keep a person young and capable of enjoying a full life as long as he lives.

In this book he not only presents a well-documented report on the value of exercise and diet but gives many specific suggestions of "how to" establish a useful fitness program.

The book is well-written, easy to read, and will be of great help to those who follow his advice. It is highly recommended.

HANS KRAUS, M.D.
Associate Professor of Physical
Medicine and Rehabilitation,
New York University

STAYING
IN THE GAME

1

What Is Aging?

> There are but three general events which happen to
> mankind: birth, life, and death. Of their birth they
> are insensible, they suffer when they die, and neglect
> to live.
>
> JEAN DE LA BRUYÈRE
> *Characters of Men*

In a billionth of a second a quark — a theoretical subatomic
particle — is old; in twice that time it has lived a lifetime and
has burned itself out, an unnoticed incident of subatomic
minutiae. The glacier plods its way through eons, planing the
rough edges off young mountains and enjoying a millennium of
respite between the granite bosoms of older ranges. The Big
Bang reverberates along Einstein's curved meridian and light
years become the physicist's milieu. Time, aside from being
the indicted "thief of youth," is the idiosyncratic referee of
history, of progress, of man's struggle with his allotted space.

How is it possible to call time idiosyncratic? What component of our existence is more constant, more dependable? We
measure the travel of radar pulses against time, and this trans-
lates into precise quantities of speed and distance. Cycles per
second, miles per hour, rotations per minute — time lends itself ideally to science, electronics, and machinery. It is only
when we attempt to measure ourselves against time that it
becomes intransigent. The reason for this is that we not only
use time as a yardstick, but we also experience it.

Children experience time differently from adults. The "lifer" in his cell experiences it differently from the lover in his or her special Eden. Sitting under the dentist's drill, for example, is likely to stretch the seconds appallingly. Time is an accurate tool for measuring the duration of just about everything but ourselves.

What is "aging," then? We ask the child at his mother's knee, "How old are you?" "Six," he replies. And this tells us something about him. He is probably cutting his six-year molars. He has recently begun school. He should be able to tie his shoelaces, and his peers, his parents, and his teachers will expect certain things of him. He will satisfy expectations to varying degrees. Yet, even at this early age he is beginning to display differences from other youngsters — with the same birthdate — in the way he is responding to aging. Unlike cheeses and fine wines, humans do not age predictably. We use time — the year — as the measure of aging because we have nothing better.

The problem takes on greater meaning a bit later in life. We begin to notice that young adults show a significant variation in the ways that aging appears to affect them. As people approach their middle years, these differences become even more pronounced, and if we observe sixty-year-olds, we find some who are laying bricks, working farms, playing tennis, or running marathons. Others are ready for, if not confined to, wheelchairs and nursing homes. Hospitals and nursing homes are overflowing with men and women in their sixties, seventies, and eighties who have become so mentally and physically deficient that they are practically nonfunctional . . . truly helpless. "Well, let's face it," one is told, "they are old . . . that's what we have to expect." Certainly, that is the way in which the disabilities associated with aging have been regarded traditionally, at least in our culture. But *is* that what we have to expect? Is that what aging means? Are the wheelchair, the rocker, the nursing home, the bedpan all we have to look forward to as we approach our later years?

As we probe the question of aging we uncover more questions. What happens to our bodies and our minds as we age? Is aging the same — or at least, a similar — experience for all of us? And now the two key questions: Is aging something that happens to us or something we do to ourselves? How much control *do* we have? If we consider the physiological effects of aging we can begin to form a strategy. *A plan for staying in the game.*

Most authorities on the subject agree that aging, as it affects the human species, has two components. The first is *primary* or *chronological aging*, and to a great extent, this type of aging is programmed into our genes. The cause of primary aging is one of the great questions — like the nature of the force of gravity — that has tantalized scientists for decades. Researchers always seem to be one step away from the big breakthrough. When two scientists associated with Cambridge University, James Watson and Francis Crick, discovered the nature of the DNA (deoxyribonucleic acid) molecule — the basic component of the chromosomes of the living cell nuclei — scientists all over the world were encouraged to believe that, at last, the secrets of chronological aging would be revealed. Aging is, after all, the death of the body's individual cells, or rather, it is their inability to continue to divide and thus regenerate the tissues of the body. In the *young body*, healthy cells are continually being produced at a rate that outpaces by far the destruction of worn-out cells. This is the time of life during which we grow. In the *mature body*, a balance of healthy cells is maintained. As cells wear out and die, they are replaced through cell division. But here's the rub: There seems to be a limit to the number of times that cells can regenerate themselves. The secrets surrounding that limit are still eluding scientists, but we do know some facts, facts that are relevant to the purposes of this book. We know that in the *aging* body the formation rate of new cells is no longer able to keep up with the demise of worn-out cells, so that degeneration of both the body and its organs occurs. We know that the chromosomes in the nucleus of each cell are programmed with all of the hereditary information that concerns us. And part of that information contains the projected life span of that cell, barring outside influences.

Barring outside influences — that's our hedge. That's what *staying in the game* is all about, because it brings us to the second type of aging: *Secondary* or *physiological aging*. This is the component of aging that we can do something about. Common sense tells us that our general health is largely determined by the way we live our lives. But there is sound evidence that much of what we call "lifestyle" has effects that reach right down into the basic structure of our bodies, right into the cell itself. *We* supply — or fail to supply — the *outside influences* that can keep cells healthy and capable of regenerating themselves for as long as possible.

Many factors affect the body, mind, and spirit as we follow our unique paths through life. If we recognize that aging — in addition to being a biological process — is a reaction to who we are, what we are, and the way in which we live our lives, then at least we know we do have some choices and more control than we suspect. Many of the world's leading authorities on aging are convinced that physical activity is the most potent weapon we can muster against the effects of aging, not only because of the direct benefits of exercise but because of the many other living habits, mind-body changes, and attitudes that seem to flow naturally from regular, rigorous, physical activity.

Recently I was introduced to Zachariah Blackestone, a well-known Washington businessman who is proprietor of the Blackestone Florist Shops, a business he started with ten dollars in capital in 1898. He distinctly remembers his first sale: 75 cents for a bouquet of roses, at 5 in the evening, after a whole day of no customers. Your mental calculator is probably questioning the date, just as mine was: 1898 . . . that's 81 years ago. Mr. Blackestone was 108 years of age on February 16, 1979. He not only goes to the office and runs a business five days a week, he also begins each day with jogging and push-ups. "I owe it all to exercise, especially jogging," says Blackestone. "When I wake up, I think I'm dead. Jogging brings my blood pressure up, and I feel like a man. I'm ready for the day."

Zachariah Blackestone has been exercising all his life. He is an outstanding example of the individual who is determined to stay in the game. Blackestone is unique in that he is and has been attuned to the factors necessary to keep him healthy and at the peak of his powers. At a time when so many people have felt only disdain for exercise and physical activity, this hearty old gentleman has got down to the basics. He is the "good animal."

Mr. Blackestone's example underscores the fact that within the human organism there are instincts that tell us what is necessary in order to enjoy a long, healthy, productive life. Some of us hear the message more clearly than others; many hear but doubt. Fewer still have been willing to act on these instincts, especially in the face of a general attitude of aversion to the physical. But now medical science, the physiologists, the specialists in aging — the same sources who used to tell people over 35 to take it easy — are in Zachariah Blackestone's camp. The circle is complete. We are now being told to return to our bodies.

In April 1975 Fredrick C. Swartz, M.D., a specialist in internal medicine and then Chairman of the Committee on Aging of the Council on Medical Service of the American Medical Association, testified before the United States Senate Subcommittee on Aging. During the course of his testimony Dr. Swartz made this observation:

> A survey of those . . . in the later years, both the well and the afflicted, reveals far too great a number who already present the shaky-hand and the tottery-gait syndrome or a tendency to go in that direction. It seems like a plague of feebleness, fragile-

ness that takes possession of the individual. . . . The free swinging gait is gone. . . . It has been said that one is old because he
.stoops, not that one stoops because he is old.

It is tragic that many Americans perceive such degeneration
as the normal consequences of aging. That it doesn't have to
be so, another prominent gerontologist has pointed out, one
has only to consider other cultures, such as African tribal
dancers who maintain slim, flexible, well-muscled bodies into
their seventies and eighties. Dr. Swartz confirms that the
treatment for the shaky-hand–tottery-gait condition is simply, "A physical exercise program, varying only in degree of
intensity."

Lawrence E. Lamb, M.D., testified before the same Senate
subcommittee as did Dr. Swartz. His comments were particu-
larly intriguing because he pointed out that so many of the
health problems, disabilities, and deterioration associated with
age are "acquired changes" rather than simply the result of
the passage of time. Because of a person's age, he or she is expected to go through these changes; so they are disregarded.
"The simple truth," said Dr. Lamb, "is that most older people
in our society are not just old. They are sick . . ."

Dr. Lamb presented another interesting idea. He suggested
that at the age of seventy a person may have reached only the
halfway mark of the possible life span. "Many of the disabilities of the seventy-year-old person," he said, "are acquired de-
fects that we have not learned to prevent or cure rather than
from time-dependent aging. The first step in managing these
problems is recognizing that they are illnesses — not just the
ravages of time."

Thinking back to the fact that aging is the result of death
of individual cells, we can appreciate the significance of Dr.
Lamb's observation that fatty deposits clog arteries and inter-
fere with circulation. Cells in the heart muscle, brain, and
other organs are deprived of oxygen and nutrients. Waste prod-
ucts and toxic substances accumulate, and the result is heart

attacks, strokes, and a multitude of other diseases. "The resulting dead heart cells, brain cells, and cells of other organs," concludes Dr. Lamb, "are dead because of a disease process, not because of time."

At this point another truth is becoming apparent: We may or may not be able to extend our life spans by the adoption of healthy living habits, but life as we live it each day is sure to be improved. The goal, then, would seem to be to maintain a healthy, vigorous, youthful body as late in life as we can. Improve the quality of each day and let the number of days take care of itself. As one wit described it: "I want to die as young as possible . . . as late in life as possible."

The first step in staying in the game is to understand that to do so requires training. Right now, each of us is engaged in a training program. Some of us are training ourselves to remain participants in the game, in some fashion, no matter how many years we may live, just like Zachariah Blackestone. Others are training themselves to drop out early, to become spectators, to retire to the sidelines with a blanket over the knees. It's never too late to change training programs, but the younger one is when the choice is made, the better the results. Coping with aging effectively is a lifetime proposition, because aging is not simply something that happens to us, it is also something we *do to ourselves.*

2

Diseases of Disuse, Diseases of Choice

The beginning of wisdom is to call things by their right names.

ANONYMOUS CHINESE PROVERB

A humorist known for his aversion to physical activity uttered the following punch line: "Lots of people I know claim that their jobs are killing them. That will never happen to me, though. You never heard of anyone resting himself to death." Now, that line probably gets its share of laughs. But, ironically, that is precisely what many people do — they literally rest themselves to death. If not to death, at least to a point of near incapacity. I refer to people who just don't want to move or exert themselves any more than is absolutely necessary. You get a strong sense of this when you pass through an airport, a bus terminal, or a department store and see droves of people ignoring staircases and lining up to use even the down escalator. These built-in habits make a strong statement about how many people feel about themselves and about using their bodies.

We Americans, as a culture, have been riding a symbolic escalator that carries us down, as we age, from one subbasement of physical degeneration to the next. Despite the fact that medical science has almost wiped out infectious diseases in America, we still get sick. We fall victim to maladies that are becoming known as "diseases of disuse and diseases of choice," ailments that are the predictable results of the way one lives one's life. Statistics dealing with the traditional definition of life expectancy are useful here since they show us how we stack up — or fail to stack up — against other societies with different lifestyles.

The life expectancy for a Caucasian woman in America is 74.9 years at birth; it is only 67.5 years for her husband. For nonwhites the figures are 67.5 years for women and 60.1 for men. Once a man reaches the age of 50 in the United States, his life expectancy is 70 years. However, on the island of Cyprus, a man of 50 can expect to live to age 83. In Iceland the figure is 79 and in Sweden, 78. Of course, these are averages, taking into account longer and shorter life spans. The point to be emphasized is that, along with the reduced life expectancies in America, we see *reduced living* before actual death. In other words, more people in America are dropping out of the game and retiring to the sidelines, waiting to die.

The major factor that makes the difference in the long-lived populations around the globe is a lifestyle that demands or encourages vigorous physical activity or regular exercise. In most of these cultures we also find that people eat foods containing less refined sugar, less saturated fat, and less salt than Americans consume. Such people usually maintain lean muscular bodies into later life, and in many of these cultures, heart attacks and strokes are practically unknown.

DISEASES OF DISUSE

It has become a cliché for health professionals to make this statement, but it has the ring of eternal truth: *If you don't use it, you lose it.* The *diseases of disuse* are the reality of that simple statement. What are they?

If any one individual can be credited with recognizing the ravages inflicted on the human body by sedentary living coupled with the stresses of our mechanized society, it is Dr. Hans Kraus. Dr. Kraus, a New York orthopedist, is an internationally regarded expert on back disabilities and a consultant to the President's Council on Physical Fitness and Sports.

In the early 1940s, Dr. Kraus and his colleague, Dr. Sonja Weber, were investigating and treating posture problems in children at Columbia-Presbyterian Hospital in New York City. They soon discovered that most of these children were basically normal but had correctable muscular deficiencies that caused posture problems. They developed a series of examinations, later known as the Kraus-Weber Test, which refined into six simple tests now used around the world not only to identify the causes of back pain but to predict its occurrence.

The most dramatic truth to emerge from the work of Doctors Kraus and Weber in the forties is that back pain and many other illnesses that plague our society are preventable. They occur from disuse of the body on one hand and the effects of stress and tension on the other.

During most of man's history, he has had to work hard even to survive. From the dawn of prehistory until fairly recent times, man has been a hunter, a farmer, and a warrior. He dealt physically with both work and danger, and like a good animal, he was endowed by nature with a special alarm system to help him respond to threatening situations. When a real or imagined threat occurs, a section of the brain called the *adrenal medula* secretes hormones that cause a figurative shift in gears, known as the "fight-flight response," and when it occurs, the body is poised for action. Respiration rate and heart rate elevate, and the blood supply to the muscles is increased. The body receives a sudden burst of energy that enables it to meet the supposed threat with physical combat or, if more prudent, with flight.

One can see how the foraging cave man, for example, was well served by the fight-flight response. The trouble is that modern living presents us with a continuous stream of stress situations. They are often job-related or associated with family or social relationships. And, although our bodies react to stress in the same way that the cave man's did, we cannot deal with it as he did. We can't fight and we can't run. Since most Americans have severely deconditioned bodies, the constant application of stressors obviously causes a multitude of stress-related diseases, among them, low-back disabilities, headaches, neck and shoulder pain, ulcers, diabetes, and heart disease.

During the early days of the American space program, NASA (the National Aeronautics and Space Administration) scientists wondered about the relationship between physical fitness and an individual's ability to handle stressful situations. They solicited help from a number of racing-car drivers who were putting their cars through practice runs for the Daytona-500 race. The drivers were wired up so that their vital functions could be monitored as they drove the course. A record was kept of each driver's pulse rate, respiration rate, body temperature, and blood pressure. The results confirmed what the physiologists had suspected all along: All of the drivers responded to hazardous situations, such as near collisions or spin-outs, in much the same way. All vital functions were elevated as a result of the fight-flight response. But the physically fit drivers returned to normal almost immediately, whereas the unfit drivers continued to experience the effects of the stress situation long after the threat had been removed. Since then, a great deal of research has been done on stress control, and it is now well established that the physically fit individual of any age is much more likely than the unfit to weather the stresses of modern living.

For a case in point as to how sedentary living and stress go hand in hand in producing diseases of disuse, it would be instructive to consider low back pain, one of the most common ailments in America. It is estimated that on any given day some seven million Americans are suffering low back disabilities. Often back problems plague an individual for a lifetime.

According to Dr. Kraus and other back specialists, it is usually a lack of muscle strength and flexibility that makes a person susceptible to this painful malady. Only a small proportion of back problems are caused by pathologies. We often hear people talking about "disk" problems, but, Dr. Kraus assures us, these are much rarer than we imagine. If we have back pain, it is much more likely to be due to muscles that are "either weak, or tense, or both." Why is this so?

Most people walk. Even the most sedentary individual has to walk to get from place to place. If he or she does absolutely no other exercise, the muscles associated with minimal locomotion are going to be used to some degree. The muscles used for walking are primarily the muscles running up the backs of the legs from the *Achilles' tendon* or heel cord, the calves of the lower legs, the hamstrings in the upper legs, and the muscles of the low back. Consequently, these muscles are stronger (and tighter) than the front muscles. Very few people have strong abdominal muscles unless they are exercising regularly. Thus, we frequently have a situation in which the muscles supporting the spine in the back are tight but the muscles in front are loose and slack.

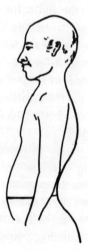

The figure in the drawing exhibits the postural defect called *lordosis,* commonly experienced by adults who are in poor physical condition. It is characterized by a protruding abdomen and a severe curve in the low back.

The illustration underscores how the spine begins to react like a flagpole with only one guy wire. The spine in the lumbar region assumes an exaggerated curve, and when this happens, it is extremely susceptible to injury and painful muscle spasms. The way to prevent low back problems is to keep the muscles both strong and resilient by performing regular exercises.

Heart disease, the leading cause of death in the United States, is a disease of disuse in many instances. We should understand that the heart is mainly a muscle, and, like any other muscle, if it is not exercised to make it stronger, it will get weaker and function less efficiently. It is not easy to isolate exercise as a simple prescription for improving heart function because there are many other factors influencing how one's heart reacts to aging, beginning with heredity and including diet, smoking and drinking habits, and the amount of stress in one's life. The most attractive feature about exercise is that its results affect other areas of function.

Consider "Bill Jones," the director of marketing for a major international corporation, a trim dynamo of a man in his early fifties. "I was about 220 pounds," said Bill, "my blood pressure was going through the roof, and my doctor told me I was a prime candidate for a heart attack or a stroke. That's when I discovered exercise." Bill Jones described how he got into a running program and over a ten-year period increased his distances. During the course of that ten years, Bill lost over fifty pounds. He stopped smoking and now only takes an occasional drink. "When I'm at a sales meeting or convention," Bill boasts, "at the end of the day I head for my running gear instead of for the cocktail lounge."

Another business executive told me a similar story. His physician had cautioned him about his weight and his high level of blood cholesterol. Just like Bill Jones, once he got into an exercise program he was able to change his lifestyle habits including smoking, drinking, and overeating in addition to bringing his blood cholesterol down to a desirable level. Exercise,

then, has proven to be an "extra point" in major lifestyle
changes that can help us avoid diseases of disuse like heart
disease and stroke.

Diseases of the muscles and joints are further examples of
what Dr. Hans Kraus has labeled "hypokinetic" diseases. These
ailments, which most people think cause limitations of movement, are diseases of disuse in the truest sense. As people age,
they are encouraged to do less and less in the way of physical
activity. Sadly, they are not even surprised to find that they
are unable to accomplish relatively simple physical tasks. They
lose their ability to play and work and often are quite resigned
to leaving the game to others.

Thanks to the pioneering work of medical men like Dr.
Kraus and Dr. Herbert DeVries, director of the Exercise and
Physiology Laboratory, Andrus Gerontology Center, University of Southern California, it is now accepted that people do
not have to lose muscle tone, strength, and range of body motion as aging occurs. The daily performance of simple exercises
can result in a fit, strong, supple body that will last for a lifetime. Dr. DeVries has reported experiments in which the aerobic capacity of individuals aged 52 to 87 was increased up to
35 percent, with commensurate improvement in muscle and
joint mobility, during the course of supervised exercise programs. One of Dr. DeVries's most exciting claims is that he is
able to take groups of men and women in their seventies, who
had been living sedentary lives, and restore them to a level of
fitness of forty-year-olds.

In his report to the Senate Subcommittee on Aging, Dr.
Raymond Harris, president of the Center for the Study of
Aging and chief of cardiology at St. Peter's Hospital in Albany,
New York, reported that ". . . more than half of the patients
who consult me complain of symptoms that they mistakenly
attribute to the aging process. However, as a geriatric cardiologist, researcher, and physician, I find that the majority of
their problems are a result of muscular and cardiovascular un-
fitness." Dr. Harris lists aches and pains of the muscles and

joints and low back strain as typical diseases of disuse.

Many physicians are now convinced that even arthritis and other diseases of the joints are more apt to be associated with disuse of the body than with regular nontraumatic use of muscles and joints as in daily rigorous exercise.

In their newsletter, *Physical Fitness Research Digest*, the President's Council on Physical Fitness and Sports listed the following physical functions or occurrences known to be associated with the aging process. However, *all* of them are greatly accelerated by sedentary living to the degree they can be truly categorized as diseases of disuse.

Heart Rate

Unless affected by exercise, little change in resting heart rate occurs during adult life. Maximum heart rate is a function of aging and is not greatly affected by exercise. Through exercise it is possible to lower the resting heart rate by 20 or 30 beats per minute. This is an excellent barometer for gauging one's increase in cardiorespiratory fitness.

Blood Pressure

Both systolic and diastolic blood pressure increase by 10 to 15 mm. Hg. (millimeters of mercury) over the span of adult life. For nonexercisers it can greatly exceed this amount.

Cardiac Output

The volume of blood passing through the heart is heavily dependent on the condition of the veins and arteries of the circulatory system. Exercisers have a definite advantage. *All* of the organs and tissues in the body of the exerciser benefit from this fact.

Respiratory Efficiency

A decline in respiratory efficiency occurs as the body ages. This decline is far more pronounced for the nonexerciser.

Aerobic Capacity

The ability of the heart and lungs to process oxygen — the aerobic capacity — is the measure of cardiorespiratory fitness. It declines with age, but, between exercisers and nonexercisers, there's no contest.

Anerobic Power

This is a measure of the body's ability to function briefly under heavy workloads. Anerobic activity can be fatal for the older nonexerciser.

Protein Synthesis

Protein synthesis is the process by which the body converts nutriments into lean muscle tissue — bulky muscle in the male, sleek muscle in the female. This process is promoted by the pituitary growth hormone and by androgen (male sex hormone) and is thus at its peak during teen years. Even in later life, individuals can build and maintain lean muscle tissue through exercise and judicious diet.

In the nonexerciser, muscle tissue, since it is not being used, gradually is replaced by fat even though an individual may be keeping his or her weight constant.

Cellular Aging

Aging of body systems takes place when active tissue, such as muscle, is replaced by metabolically less active tissue, such as fat. Exercise and prudent diet retard this process.

Muscular Strength

Unless enhanced by exercise, muscular strength peaks at about age 17. Muscles that are used will maintain their strength levels until about age 45, then decline about 15 percent over the next 20 years. With vigorous exercise, it is possible to increase strength levels at almost any time in one's life and even to forestall, to some degree, the expected 15 percent decline from maximum levels.

*

Thomas K. Cureton, director of the Physical Fitness Institute at the University of Illinois, is a well-recognized researcher and activist in adult physical fitness. In his book *The Physiological Effects of Exercise Programs on Adults* he makes these points:

a. Men — even young men — are not doing enough vigorous exercise to keep the blood flowing through the muscles in adequate amounts, an important key to physical fitness. Thus, physiological aging comes upon modern man with astonishing rapidity, especially those who are sedentary.

b. In the trained state the nervous system is prepared for action rather than inaction. In general, the individual is trained away from persistent sedentary tendencies and toward a higher sympathetic and ragus tone leading toward a desire for physical activity.

The evidence is in on sedentary living and its relationship to diseases of disuse. The latest research proves that even bone degeneration, long thought to be a consequence of aging, is another result of inactivity. Physically active people are going to take strong, resilient bones into old age with them. Sedentary folk are going to have frail, fragile bones. Muscles that are weak and slack, hanging on fragile bones, simply can't hold the body together properly. Internal organs are not supported — aside from suffering from inadequate circulation — so they get sick.

Even senility (and what disease has been more firmly associated with aging?) is now being dealt with as a disease of disuse. Older persons who are underexercised, with resultant poor circulation to the brain, who rarely receive intellectual stimulation or challenges, who are expected to show a reduction in cognitive capability, eventually make that a self-fulfilling prophecy. When these same older people exercise daily, eat properly, and experience a measure of mental stimuli, they often return to previous levels of mental capacity.

DISEASES OF CHOICE

It now becomes more obvious that aging is, indeed, something that we do to ourselves. The *diseases of choice* underscore that reality. These ailments, which accelerate the aging process, often overlap with the previously discussed diseases of disuse. They are diseases that are related to our conscious lifestyle habits, and they have direct, predictable effects on health.

Smoking is, of course, the most insidious habit of modern man, especially since very few people really want to do it. A curse for those who smoke, it is becoming increasingly offensive to those who do not. It has no redeeming social value, and it is a major contributing factor in heart disease, circulatory diseases, lung and throat cancer, such respiratory diseases as emphysema, and malignancies of many types. Dr. Kenneth Cooper, the famed author and director of the Aerobics Fitness Center in Dallas, Texas, says flatly, "You cannot smoke and be fit."

Alcohol abuse is right up there with smoking as a major health problem. We are all familiar with the consequences of alcoholism and with the so-called "problem drinker," but few people are aware of the collateral damage being done to the body through habitual dependence on alcohol. Such damage includes destruction of brain cells, cirrhosis of the liver, heart damage, and elevation of serum cholesterol. It is common for the heavy user of alcohol to appear to age far more rapidly than his or her contemporaries.

Overeating is a characteristic problem of our culture that, in turn, breeds many of the diseases of choice: Diabetes, high blood pressure, heart and artery disease are just a few ailments resulting from what and how much we eat. As everyone with an eating problem knows, these problems are not easy to deal with. Almost all of the diseases of choice involve one or more lifestyle habits that many individuals have found difficult or impossible to eliminate. One of the reasons for this is that we are very complex beings, and everything we are and everything we do is reflected in and interrelates with everything else we are and everything else we do. It's important to know this. Psychologists dealing with behavior modification are learning that the best way to eliminate bad habits is to embrace good ones. The admonitions of physicians, family, and friends — the "you shouldn'ts" and the "you mustn'ts" — have never been really effective at getting people to change lifestyle habits. It's a matter of putting a positive factor such as exercise into our lives and making it a personal choice. Then many other problems begin to take care of themselves.

3
Stress and Aging

My soul is a broken field ploughed by pain
SARA TEASDALE
The Broken Field

There are many factors involved in aging and many theories as
to what these factors are. *Staying in the Game* is concerned
with the factors over which we have some control. Stress falls
into that category. The effects, both physiological and psychological, of stress are now recognized as playing a major role in
both general health and aging. One of the most pronounced
effects of our high-technology, competitive society is the bruis-
ing stress factors it imposes on us. But what is stress? Is it all
bad? How does it affect us, and what can we do about it?

Stress is a psychophysiological reaction to the people, ob-
jects, and events surrounding us; it is our reaction to changes
in our environment. *Stressors* are the specific incidents that
cause us to experience a stress reaction. Not all stress is harm-
ful. Without stress we wouldn't be motivated. We all have
ambitions and responsibilities that prod us into action, and
that action satisfies the stress response. It is only when the
stressors impose demands upon us that we cannot satisfy, or
when they come too quickly, that we begin to have problems.

Behavioral scientists describe the stress response in terms
of a characteristic common to both men and animals. It is
called the "fight-flight response."

What about you? You are continually assaulted with threatening situations: The mortgage payment may be overdue; your daughter may need braces; the boss may have it in for you; perhaps you or a loved one is threatened by a serious illness. Your mind/body system responds to these situations in the same way an animal's does. Remember, man was once primarily a hunter and a fighter, and the fight or flight response was necessary to help him survive life-threatening situations. Whenever you become aware of something that poses a danger to your health, your safety, your self-esteem, your job, your social position, or your financial security, you experience the fight or flight response. Unfortunately, in most situations we can neither fight nor flee. You can't respond to the boss with a karate chop when he tells you your sales figures are off, and you can't run away and hide either. There's no way to fight back against inflation, which may be eating away at a pension or other fixed income, and you can't flee from that problem. What happens is that each of the life situations that poses a threat causes an alarm reaction. We all know how that feels. The heart pounds, and we feel very keyed up. Sleep becomes difficult or impossible. The body has been prepared for action that has been denied. Theoretically, when the threatening situation is removed, the mind/body system returns to a pre-stress state. But many of the problems that we find threatening don't go away. Further, in our complex society, stressful events may occur at such a rapid pace that one may never achieve a pre-stress state ... at least not for very long. It is becoming evident that the result of continual stress, of living with an endless succession of alarm reactions, is illness, often manifested by symptoms associated with aging.

Dr. Hans Selye of the University of Toronto is considered the world's leading authority on stress. Dr. Selye has established definite links between stress and aging. He believes that individuals can take only so much stress before the organism begins to break down and wear out. Researchers like Dr. Kenneth Pelletier have established convincing evidence that stress is a factor — perhaps the decisive factor — in such maladies as cardiovascular disease, arthritis, respiratory illness, cancer, low back disabilities, and nervous disorders. Dr. Pelletier's research has convinced him that people of all ages are affected by stress, but these effects, being cumulative, may not show up until the forties or fifties. At that time it is natural to blame aging for the things going wrong in the body. "Stress disorders," says Dr. Pelletier, "are based upon the slow developmental accumulation of psychological and physical stress responses throughout the life of the individual."

When we become aware of stress factors, we see that they are everywhere. Pollution of the environment — our air, food, and water — causes stress; high noise levels cause stress; overcrowding, job pressures, social relationships, boredom, all cause stress. Then, why isn't everyone affected equally? Why don't we all suffer the effects of stress and tension? Well, many of us do. Cardiovascular disease will kill over half a million people this year in our country. Cancer deaths are not far behind, and on any given day, over 7 million Americans will be sidelined by low back pain. If we accept the premise that these diseases are — at least to some degree — caused by stress, then we can see that stress and its effects are, indeed, affecting many of us. Some people seem to handle stress better than others. They are the people who avoid the stress-related maladies. Since *Staying in the Game* is about fighting back, let's see how we can do this.

Dr. David Munz, a psychologist associated with the Center for the Application of Behavioral Science at St. Louis University, describes how some people attempt to handle stress. "People under stress often experience physiological symptoms. This causes fear, so the stress intensifies." Under these circumstances, the individual often resorts to alcohol, smoking, overeating, or drugs. Of course, these "remedies" further deteriorate the body. So what we end up with is a "feedback loop" of anxiety, mental and physical distress, and remedies that feed that distress. As this closed system intensifies, various kinds of illness can result. What we have to do is break the loop.

The best way to begin coping with stress is to try to remove some of the stressful situations from our lives. Of course, it just isn't possible to eliminate everything from our lives that will cause stress and tension, but it is important to know just what the stressors in our lives are. It is also important to understand that even "good" occurrences can be stressful if they require major adjustments. Quantitatively, events vary in terms of their effect on one's physiology. Two psychiatrists from the University of Washington Medical School, Dr. Thomas H. Holmes and Dr. Richard H. Rahe, have taken Dr. Selye's theory concerning the cumulative effects of stress one step further by designing a scale of stressful situations. They call this list of life situations "The Social Readjustment Scale." The numerical value next to each life event represents the average value assigned to that event by several hundred individuals interviewed by Dr. Holmes and Dr. Rahe.

STRESS VERSUS LIFE EVENTS

Events	*Impact*
Death of spouse	100
Divorce	73
Marital separation	65
Jail term	63
Death of close family member	63
Personal injury or illness	53
Marriage	50
Fired at work	47
Marital reconciliation	45
Retirement	45
Change in health of family member	44
Pregnancy	40
Sex difficulties	39

Events	Impact
Gain of new family member	39
Business readjustment	39
Change in financial state	38
Death of close friend	37
Change to different line of work	36
Change in number of arguments with spouse	35
Mortgage over $10,000	31
Foreclosure of mortgage or loan	30
Change in responsibilities at work	29
Son or daughter leaving home	29
Trouble with in-laws	29
Outstanding personal achievement	28
Wife begins or stops work	26
Begin or end school	26
Change in living conditions	25
Revision of personal habits	24
Trouble with boss	23
Change in working hours or conditions	20
Change in residence	20
Change in schools	20
Change in recreation	19
Change in church activities	19
Change in social activities	18
Mortgage or loan less than $10,000	17
Change in sleeping habits	16
Change in number of family get-togethers	15
Change in eating habits	15
Vacation	13
Christmas	12
Minor violations of the law	11

Paul T. Costa, Jr., Ph.D., chief psychologist at the Gerontology Center at the National Institute of Aging in Baltimore, Maryland, insists that age is not a factor in an individual's ability to cope with stressful events. What is significant is one's personality and the way one feels about himself or herself and these events. No event — of itself — can cause an alarm reaction to occur. It is necessary for the individual to assess the event and interpret it as threatening. Thus, one positive step one can take to defuse some stressful situations is to reassess these situations; one can try to analyze just exactly what is causing the anxiety and then determine if that anxiety is justified. Worrying can become a habit. It doesn't solve the problem but makes it worse by inhibiting the ability to deal with it.

I recently had a discussion with a married woman who works as an administrative assistant in a medium-sized company. Because of market conditions, the company had laid off several employees. The woman told me that she had been "worrying herself sick" over the possibility that she, too, might lose her job. A conversation with a clergyman caused her to re-evaluate her job situation. "He asked me to be specific about what I was anxious about," she said. "Would we starve? No, of course not. Would we lose our home? No, my husband's income was adequate to cover all necessities." The clergyman pointed out that the worst thing that could happen would be that things would be tight for a while until she found another job — maybe even a better one. So the challenge is to meet stressful situations head-on; pick them apart to see what is causing anxiety. At that point we can decide: First, is the situation really worth worrying about? Second, how can we deal with it to remove it as a stressor?

Now, we won't be able to remove all stress situations in this manner, but, if we eliminate some, we are that much ahead of the game. What about the effects of the remaining stressful events in our lives? How does one fight back? Well, the behavioral scientists have come up with what might be called a "double play" combination to offset the effects of stress. The two weapons we can all employ are (1) exercise and (2) relaxation. A sport, being play, combines both of these elements. Dr. Kathryn Cramer, executive director of the Center for the

Application of Behavioral Science, explained how exercise helps an individual to cope with stress. "Modern life," said Dr. Cramer, "imposes a continual barrage of ambiguous stress upon most of us. We really don't know all of the reasons why we are tense and anxious. When we exercise we substitute a specific physical stress for all of the ambiguous mental stress. Then, when we remove that physical stress, we can return to a pre-stress condition."

Perhaps, one of the reasons that the physically fit person handles stress well can be related to what we learned earlier about the fight or flight response. If the stresses of modern living prepare the body for action, our daily exercise activities — our training programs — provide that action. The body is turned loose; the requirement for movement is satisfied; nervous energies are burned off.

The other half of our one-two punch against stress is relaxation. Some health professionals and health writers are emphasizing exercise as the best way to combat stress; others are big on relaxation. But exercise and relaxation needn't be an either-or choice because they work so well together. In fact, you really can't separate them. One of the first things you will notice when you begin exercise and recreational sports is that you can relax more easily and completely. Conversely, relaxation makes you a better athlete.

One of the most dramatic examples of how relaxation can be employed as an antidote for stress-related maladies is in the treatment of hypertension (high blood pressure). Clinicians using biofeedback instruments are showing hypertensive patients how to bring their blood pressure down by "willing" it down. Transcendental Meditation and other relaxation techniques are now available just about everywhere at clinics, Ys, and adult education classes. Readers who feel that they have a special problem with inability to relax are urged to consider taking a relaxation class as an adjunct to their exercise programs. Most readers, however, will be able to apply the following simple procedures developed by the Department of Health Promotion at St. Louis University Medical Center:

DEEP ABDOMINAL BREATHING
FOR RELAXATION

Objective

To demonstrate and practice deep breathing as a relaxation skill and as a stress-reaction intervention. To demonstrate and explain the interrelationship of physiological patterns and psychological states. To introduce the concept of consciously and purposefully controlling a simple physiological pattern.

Procedure
Part I — Posture

1. Stand in a comfortable position with the feet a little more than shoulder width apart, knees straight but not locked.
2. The arms hang loosely at the sides, and the shoulders should be relaxed.
3. Even though the body is relaxed, good posture is maintained; the joints are straight but not locked, firm but not stiff. The difference between straight and locked joints is easily noticed at the elbows. Observe the position of the knee joint, which should also have just a slight bend and should not be locked tightly.
4. The head is held up and level, with the neck relaxed.

Part II — Chest Breathing

1. Many people breathe from the chest, with the upper part of the chest lifting.
2. The proper hingelike movement of the sternum contrasted with the improper up-and-down movement of chest breathing is easily noticed by placing the palm of one hand on the breastbone and the other hand on the stomach. Observe the difference

in the movement patterns of chest breathing versus abdominal breathing.

3. Various psychological states have associated breathing patterns; for example, demonstrate for yourself the rapid shallow breathing pattern common during anxiety reactions.

4. Conscious control of breathing patterns will, in turn, facilitate the associated psychological state. Learning a deep relaxed breath is useful in maintaining a relaxed, though very active, mind.

Part III — Deep Abdominal Breathing

1. When people are very relaxed or asleep, breath is drawn from lower in the abdomen. This is a more natural, more efficient pattern.

2. The chest should be relaxed and the ribs allowed to move naturally. As the diaphragm moves downward on breathing in, the "stomach" will move outward; therefore, the gut should be allowed to "hang out." This is the opposite of what our culture encourages as in the expression "stomach in, chest out."

3. Close your eyes and practice deep abdominal breathing for about ten or more cycles. The pace should be slow and natural, not at all rushed. Breathe in only when you feel the need and take in only as much air as is comfortable.

4. Before opening your eyes, notice any change in your mental state, even if very slight. Learning control over and understanding of the mind and body begins by observing the little changes one can produce.

INTEGRATION EXERCISE: RELAXATION OF THE LUMBAR SPINE

Objective

To reset the tone in the muscles attached to the lower spine in order to allow a greater degree of relaxation and to increase comfort while you are lying on your back (supine) on the floor.

Procedure
Part I — Crossing the Legs

1. Lie flat on your back on the floor and notice any discomfort in the low back. With either hand feel the space between the floor and the lower back.
2. Lift the knees so the feet rest flat on the floor.
3. The arms lie comfortably a little less than 90° from the side of the body.
4. Lift the right leg over the left so the legs are crossed with the right knee resting near the left.
5. Take in a deep breath from the lower abdomen. As this breath is released the legs are allowed to drop to the right, pulled by gravity into a comfortable stretch.
6. Once the breath is exhaled, pause a short moment and relax. Notice the stretch through the hip to the shoulder.
7. With the next inhalation, the legs are brought back up to the center as in step 4.
8. Repeat 5 to 10 times. Switch leg positions and repeat to the other side.
9. Allow the knees to drop to the side. Slowly extend the legs to lie flat on the floor. Notice any changes in the relationship of your body to the ground, especially the arch in the lower back.

Part II — Folding the Hands

1. Lift both arms straight above the chest and clasp the fingers together.
2. Notice the triangle formed by the arms on each side and the shoulders and chest at the base. This triangle is to be maintained throughout this section of the exercise.
3. Lift the knees and rest the feet flat on the floor.
4. Take in a deep breath from the lower abdomen and, while exhaling, lean the entire "triangle" to the right. With this movement the left shoulder will be gently pulled off the floor. Notice the stretch from the shoulder to the hip.

5. Inhale naturally and bring the arms back to the central position.

6. Repeat 5 to 10 times, then continue to the other side (from steps 4 to 6).

Part III — Close

1. With the arms back to the central position, unfold the hands and allow the elbows to slowly touch the floor. The forearms are then allowed to gently return to the floor.

2. Once again allow the knees to fall to the side and extend the legs slowly back to the floor.

3. Notice the new relationship of the body to the floor.

4. At this point, you may wish to record your observations or proceed directly into another exercise for a deeper experience of relaxation (i.e., progressive relaxation).

PROGRESSIVE RELAXATION

Objectives

To allow the release of muscular tension in all parts of the body. To increase the awareness of the experience of relaxing a muscle group while simultaneously increasing conscious control over a greater number of muscle groups.

Procedure

1. Assume a comfortable position. This exercise may be done lying down.

2. This is a method of learning to relax by increasing tension. The sensation experienced when the tension is *released* should be noticed and emphasized. Releasing of tension is the skill to be learned.

3. Identify the feet as the first area to tense. The tension is to last about 6 to 8 seconds with each muscle group.

4. Tense the feet . . . tense . . . *Tense* . . . TENSER . . . hold . . . and relax.

5. And now, tense the calves . . . tense . . . tighter . . . tenser . . . and relax.

6. ... the thighs ...

7. ... the buttocks ...

8. ... the lower abdomen and pelvis ...

9. ... the small of the back ...

10. ... the upper back ...

11. ... the stomach ...

12. ... the chest ...

13. ... the shoulders ...

14. ... the arms ...

15. ... the neck ...

16. ... the face ... "the uglier the better" ...

17. ... the frontalis ... (the muscle that wrinkles the forehead and is associated with stress and mental tension) ...

18. ... the occipitalis (the muscle in the back of the head) ... The occipitalis may be hard for some people to identify and tense. This is a good example of the process of consciously tensing a muscle in order to become familiar with that muscle. It is through this familiarity that enough control can be learned to allow a person to deliberately relax.

19. ... and now the whole body ...

20. Relax and search inwardly for any tense muscles. If any are found, these should be tensed and released.

21. Notice any sensations of heaviness or relaxation and observe the changes that have taken place in the body.

4

The Food Problem

Other men live to eat, while I eat to live.

SOCRATES

For many of us, the act of eating is a problem. According to some estimates, up to 80 percent of American men and women are overweight. Obesity is not compatible with the goals that we are laying out for ourselves for staying in the game, but a reader should not be intimidated by a weight problem. We are going to take an entirely new approach, one that will not require making any drastic changes in eating habits, at least not at the outset.

The task is to mobilize our eating as a force to help us move toward our fitness and growth goals. And that's really not so difficult. First of all, we should recognize that any behavior pattern, like eating, is intimately linked with everything else we do and everything that we are. An individual who has become sedentary, who does nothing physical, who is growing softer and plumper and visibly older every day is not in the proper frame of mind to modify his or her eating patterns in a meaningful and permanent way. Such a person is likely to resort to crash diets or fad diets from time to time. We are not going to even mention the word *diet* again because it implies a temporary measure to which one resorts for a predetermined period of time, after which the dieter ends the diet and returns to his or her former eating habits. It seldom, if ever, works over the long term. What we are going to do is to capitalize on the fact that we are committed to growth (in every respect except waist measurement) and put all of our growth factors together. Here's how it works. We are employing exercise and physical activity as the "entry point" into our fitness/growth program; so, right away, we are ahead of the game. Before we even think about how we can modify food intake, we will be chipping away at body fat by virtue of increased daily calorie burn. Depending on the intensity of your exercise program, you will be burning between several hundred and a couple of thousand calories each week. And each time you can chalk off 3,500 calories expended in exercise, you've burned away a pound of fat.

As an exerciser you have a psychological factor working for you also. I'm a morning jogger, for example. I go out for my morning run sometime between 5:30 and 7:30 A.M. Now, that takes a certain amount of resolution and discipline, especially when the bed is warm and cozy on a cold winter morning. That, together with half an hour to an hour out on the road, is an investment. I feel as though I've done something worthwhile. There's no way that I'm going to dump a stack of pancakes or waffles down on top of that. At that point, it's not even a case of will power; it simply would be inconceivable to blow my investment on a high-calorie breakfast. So, as your exercise and physical activity program begins to take shape, you'll find that you will be making automatic little accommodations in your eating habits that might be described as a "show of respect" for your physical investment.

You may expect to be hungrier once you begin exercising regularly, but usually that is not the case. Once again, the psychophysiology of the exercise is going to come to your rescue. You may be ravenously hungry before going out for a run or a brisk walk. But once you elevate your respiration and heart rates and break into a light sweat, you'll notice that the hungry feeling gradually disappears. After your workout, you may not feel like eating at all. What has happened is that your blood sugar level has been elevated due to your physical activity. This is a signal to your brain that it is a time for energy expenditure rather than food intake. So, your appetite regulating mechanism shuts your appetite down for a while.

Another phenomenon takes place in the body of the exerciser that concerns the quality rather than quantity of the food he or she eats. As the individual becomes more of a physical creature the body itself begins to reject empty calories, foods that undermine the physical, foods that contribute nothing. Food preferences change, very gradually, very subtly, until a highly nutritious low calorie menu is the preferred one. Controlled experiments confirm this, and many athletes comment on this shift, especially distance runners. Joggers and even dedicated walkers insist that they experience a gradual orientation toward the foods that can play a positive role in their bodies' reorientation toward the physical.

Now, none of the above aids to weight control are available to the person who simply "diets." Our program begins with exercise and allows the benefits of exercise to radiate out into all of the other aspects of life. If divesting your body of fat is necessary, your exercise program is already at work at that problem, and there are other things you can do. The simplest, at first, is to give up *one* food or treat voluntarily each day. This should be a food, a drink, or a dessert that contributes little or nothing to your nutrition. Now, that's not a drastic lifestyle change; it's one anyone can handle. But the results can be staggering. Let's look at an example. Suppose, for example, that Betty decides to take a brisk walk for one hour, five times a week. Betty will expend approximately 1400 calories per week through her walking, alone. Now if Betty eliminates just one piece of apple pie or its equivalent each day, that's another 2100 calories — even if we allow her to have her piece of pie on Sunday. Betty has established a *calorie deficit* of 3500 calories a week. That's equivalent to a pound of fat. Betty can lose about 50 pounds of fat over the course of a year at that rate. Better than any crash diet, and it's a long-term weight loss with only good side effects. Betty's friends will tell her that she looks years younger.

It's the combination of diet and exercise which gives us a "one-two" punch against body fat. Experience indicates that it is better to start with exercise and recreational sports. When these physical activities become an important part of your life, other lifestyle changes will result. Perhaps, the stress reduction effects of your exercise program will modify your need to eat or drink compulsively. Many joggers and folks who do other types of exercise regularly find that the disciplines called upon to stick to the exercise program can be applied to other components of their fitness/growth experience, such as eating, drinking, or smoking habits.   2095072

Just as important as *how much we eat* is *what we eat*. Once we approach the nutrition question, we discover a good deal of controversy. But certain facts are emerging as basic truths in terms of nutrition and general good health. The foods that are deleterious to good health often seem to accelerate aging, as well. For the sake of brevity and simplicity, here are seven important points:

1. Fatty foods are not healthful. They contribute to obesity, may be a factor in cardiovascular disease, and there is some evidence that they contribute to the aging of the cells and the development of some forms of cancer.

2. Refined sugar has no nutritional value. It contributes to obesity, hypoglycemia, emotional instability, and behavioral problems. It is addictive and impedes the metabolism of fats.

3. Excessive salt in the diet causes high blood pressure and retention of fluids, with attendant problems such as edema and excess weight.

4. Artificial substances like chemical preservatives, flavorings, and colorings are pollutants and may be the cause of far

more health problems than we now attribute to them. They should be avoided.

5. Many processed foods, in addition to being laced with artificial coloring, flavoring, and preservatives, have been stripped of their nutriments.

6. Some nutritionists insist that vitamin and mineral supplements — especially vitamins C and E and the mineral selinium — help prevent oxidation and aging of the body cells.

7. Alcohol destroys brain cells, damages the liver, contributes to heart disease, and speeds up aging. (There is evidence, on the other hand, that a couple of ounces of wine each day increase the possibility of longevity, apparently by reducing the percentage of low density lipoproteins in the blood.)

What should you eat? It is estimated that about 20 percent of our food intake should be protein, which contains the amino acids our bodies require for maintenance and repair of cells. You can see that this is vitally important in forestalling the aging of the body. It's one of the reasons why people subjected to poor diets and malnutrition often look years older than their chronological ages. Certain types of protein sources contain all of the essential amino acids, and these are called "complete" proteins. The best sources for complete proteins are meat, milk, eggs, yogurt, and most cheeses. Most vegetable sources of protein are incomplete (soy beans are the exception) although taken in the right combinations all of the amino acids may be present.

That's why we hear so much about a "balanced diet." If we try to obtain all of our protein from meat and dairy sources, we ingest too much animal fat. So the vegetable sources are just as important, although it is not advised to rely totally on them. Beans, peas, lentils, corn, and cereal grains are fine sources of protein as well as being rich in other nutriments. Fresh fruits and vegetables and green, leafy vegetables round out what we think of as a balanced diet.

Many readers will want to give serious attention to what

and how much they eat. Such a detailed program is beyond the scope of this book, but I strongly encourage interest in nutrition, and I have included in the Bibliography two books that I highly recommend to help the reader stay in the game, one being *Psychodietetics*, by Cheraskin, Ringsdorf, and Brecker, and the other, *The Pritikin Program for Diet and Exercise.*

5

Rediscovering the Athlete Within Us

> The weakest among us can become some kind of athlete, but only the strongest can survive as spectators. Only the hardiest can withstand the perils of inertia, inactivity, and immobility. Only the most resilient can cope with the squandering of time, the deterioration of fitness, the loss of creativity, the frustration of the emotions, and the dulling of the moral sense that can afflict the dedicated spectator.
>
> GEORGE SHEEHAN

In his book on the mind/body relationship and the joy of living life physically, *The Ultimate Athlete*, George Leonard invites each reader to embark on a mystical excursion in search of the athlete hidden within him. He begins with this evocative statement:

> The athlete that dwells within each of us is more than an abstract ideal. It is a living presence that can change the way we feel and live. Searching for our inner athlete may lead us into sports and regular exercise and thus to the health promised by the physical fitness organizations — and that may be justification enough. But what I have in mind goes beyond fitness; it involves entering the realms of music and poetry, of the turning of the planets, of the understanding of death.

Much of the writing dealing with physical fitness and allied subjects — and I refer to the literature, not merely the how-to texts — is being written by writers in their forties and fifties who discovered fitness rather late in life. The literature is emerging because such individuals such as George Leonard, Jim Fixx, Hal Higdon, Dr. Thaddeus Kostrubala, and Dr. George Sheehan found more than heightened physical energies when they resurrected their athlete-selves. It was an entry point into a new physical-mental-spiritual symbiosis. Cardiologist/marathon runner/philosopher George Sheehan, author of the best seller *Running and Being*, speaks of the total transformation possible to the man or woman who returns to the body.

> The definition of an athlete [says Sheehan] is someone attempting to get the most from his or her genetic endowment by training in the environment. The reborn athlete begins to understand that, like David, he, too, is marvelously made whether or not he is quite up to being a Joe Namath or an O. J. Simpson. And each of us [he insists] can be an athlete.

One need not be a writer to wax eloquent when the dormant athlete emerges. A story in *Time* magazine (June 26, 1978) quotes Carolyn Bravakis, a Connecticut housewife: "All my life I never did anything. The only time I went outside was to hang the wash." One could make a fair case for typecasting Carolyn Bravakis as the typical American homemaker: sedentary in her living habits except for household chores, putting on a few pounds each year, slowly coming apart at the seams physically. But Carolyn was fortunate enough to encounter a challenge that would change not only her lifestyle but her very being. Her brother organized a 10,000-meter race and persuaded her to enter. When she became exhausted halfway through the race and had to quit, she was faced with a decision. She would either have to accept the fact that for her it was going to be downhill from then on as far as her physical being was concerned, or she would have to make a serious commitment to get herself together physically. "I was so dis-

gusted with myself," she said, "that I began to run seriously."
One year later, in 1977, she finished 29th among women runners in the Boston Marathon; in 1978 she finished number 12.
Carolyn Bravakis sums up the effect of her running on her
life this way: "I have more self-confidence, more energy than
I had before. And when I run in the rain, I feel like a six-year-
old."

The six-year-old, of course, knows these things instinctively.
She dwells happily and comfortably within her body and is,
according to the physiologists, the most nearly perfect human
machine. She literally radiates energy.

Think about your own childhood. Almost every memory
from your early youth will be, no doubt, an adventure in motion. Swimming, climbing trees, learning to dive, the first
experimental steps on skis or ice skates. These are the mem-
ories that endure from childhood.

George Sheehan echoes Emerson's admonition that we become "good animals." Very young children understand this.
It is only when we become old enough to "reason" that such
factors as fashion, custom, and whatever happens to be "in"
begin to govern our actions, and our animal nature becomes
disreputable. Watch very young children. They run and skip
and tumble with the same innocent abandon displayed by
month-old lion cubs. The lioness patiently ignores the horse-
play and allows her babies to play. The cub develops. A major
difference in the play of the young human and that of the
lion or tiger cub is that the human child knows that he or she
is playing. And while the running and racing, the rough-
housing and the mock battles of childhood may once have
been nature's way of preparing man for his role as meat eater
and hunter and sometime warrior, these playful pursuits may
mean for modern man simply the gratification of an instinct
to keep the physical dimension in the picture. It is precisely
at this moment, though, that the process of splitting off from
our bodies often begins, a process that often starts in the

home. Many adults, especially those who have succeeded at suppressing in themselves the ability — alas, even the desire — to move, tend to be put off and annoyed by movement taking place around them. How often we hear parents exhorting their children to "stop that infernal running!" The active child is, too often, urged to sit down and watch TV or engage in some similarly dynamic pursuit.

For many of us — those of us in our thirties, forties, fifties, and older — the athlete within us was buried by the time we left childhood. This can happen for a number of reasons.

One explanation for why so many of us have become separated from our inner athlete is that those in charge of our lives often succeed in taking the fun out of movement. Consider what happened to most of us in school, especially in high school and college: We were herded into physical education classes. As a group, physical education teachers are not necessarily at fault. Much of the negative backwash from physical education or "PT" is a result of some deep-rooted cultural aberrations rather than a lack of dedication or professionalism among phys. ed. teachers. By virtue of the wisdom of western education and because of its largely compulsory status, practically every child in America learned to classify his or her physical dimension — the running, jumping, climbing, and tumbling, the actions that had been a spontaneous, natural joy — under the scholastic umbrella that educators are so fond of calling *work*. First period . . . Math. Second period . . . English. Third period . . . PT. Everyone line up . . . two minutes of jumping jacks. Thus, physical activity is reduced to the monotony of the multiplication table. Why, inquires George Leonard, didn't they ever try to teach us that using our bodies and developing our bodies could feel good? Why didn't they teach us how good it could feel to be fit and strong? We heard a great deal about *mens sana in corpore sano*, but no one listened. *A sound mind in a sound body*. These words just didn't register in any meaningful way, at least not then.

No one translated them into the basic acceptable truth: that the *me* I was designed to be is a physical *me*, a mental *me*, and a spiritual *me*, and to maximize any member of this trinity it is necessary to maximize the others.

And while the guns are trained on the hypothetical "they" — one more salvo: Why did they teach us that exercise is punishment?

Perhaps the most insidious enemy of the *inner athlete* is acceptance of the idea that exercise is punishment. From the academic world to the military establishment, a favorite device of coaches, phys. ed. instructors, and drill sergeants is to build an association between exercise (i.e., pushups, running laps, etc.) and pain and punishment as a means of enforcing discipline. Show up late for gym class or football practice, and it's ten laps around the field. A speck of dirt in the barrel of your rifle in Marine Corps boot camp might cost you a hundred pushups.

This association — exercise/pain/punishment — usually affects people negatively, sometimes rather strangely. Recently, I participated in a radio talk show in Atlanta to discuss my book *Shape Up for Sports*, a manual of exercises and conditioning activities for the weekend athlete. It was a listener-participation show, and one listener who called in typified the "muscle head" mentality. The caller was angered by the fact that many of the books dealing with fitness and running frequently made reference to the fact that a rhythmic, endurance-type exercise could, for some people, be a joyful, mind-expanding experience. "Now, I'm fifty years old," the bombastic gentleman shouted, "and I've run several miles every day since I got out of the army when I was twenty-one. And . . . damn it! Running is work . . . hard work. I do it because it's good for me, but there's nothing mind blowing about it."

Now, this radio listener in Atlanta obviously requires the feeling that he is doing something punishing and difficult and painful. It makes him feel more worthy as a person to *endure* his daily penitential rite because, as he said, "it's good for me." It angers him to read or hear that the figurative "hairshirt" he wears is a joyful experience for someone else. He is not about to believe it.

Of course, many of the people who have been subjected to the exercise-as-punishment treatment simply forsake exercise forever. Then, there are others who have the desire to rehabilitate themselves physically. They will perhaps have to learn to experience exercise as a form of play in order to erase the punishment image.

The third pressure point our culture brings to bear on our inner athletes is the notion that, if one couldn't make the varsity ... if one couldn't be a super star, then one should be a *watcher* instead of a *doer*. Here again, the academic environment was the main culprit. Sports was the thing. Every kid was going to make the team. It didn't take us very long to find out that many of us weren't going to make any team. A freshman basketball team, for example, that carried only 10 players had to say no to perhaps 100 or more other boys. The girls had a similar problem. High schools and colleges built their athletic programs around team sports. Everyone else was expected to buy tickets and "support the team." Until recently, not much thought was given to creating extensive athletic programs for all students.

So we joined the ranks of the spectators, and our milieu became the grandstand. Our inner athlete was benched.

*

Fortunately, things are beginning to change, and many of today's youngsters are being exposed to more positive programs of physical activity. Instead of the *pain/punishment* association, many schools are implementing creative approaches to physical education. These take into account the individual student's somatotype (body type), his or her psychological

disposition regarding individual or team sports, with the goal
being to establish a *fun/play/pleasure* association. Lifetime
sports rather than team sports are being stressed.

One of the exciting facts emerging from the new physical
education — and this has ramifications for all of us, no matter
what age we may be — is that there is a definite correlation
between physical activity, physical fitness, and one's creative
and cognitive capabilities. We've always suspected that by
being fit we could accomplish all of our tasks — physical and
cerebral — more happily and more efficiently. That this is
true is now being proven in ways and to degrees we hadn't
imagined.

In one experiment reported by the President's Council on
Physical Fitness and Sports in their publication, *Physical Fitness Research Digest*, a freshman prep-school class was divided
into two groups, experimental and control groups with com-
parable intelligence quotients. The experimental group participated in physical fitness activities two mornings per week
and the control group did not. The results were the following:
The general academic average of the experimental group improved in relation to that of the control group. The number
of honor grades improved for the experimental group in com-
parison to the control group. The number of failing grades
decreased for the experimental group and increased for the
control group.

Another impressive study was conducted at the University
of Marburg in Germany. Physiologists there repeatedly tested
the concentration of 300 children nine to twelve years of age.
The testing procedure was preceded each time by either a
gymnastics class or a biology lesson. The children's average
power of concentration was about 12 percent higher after the
gymnastics class than after the biology class. This outcome was
even more decisive (23 percent higher after gymnastics) when
a mathematics examination was given in place of the concentration test.

Parallel experiments were conducted in academies in Vanves,

France, and in Brussels, Belgium. Experimental groups had their academic studies reduced by two or more hours per day, with a corresponding increase in the amount of time devoted to physical improvement. A general improvement in physical fitness occurred; however, there was also an increase in academic achievement. For example, the control group in the Vanves experiment achieved an average of 78 percent in pursuit of the elementary study certificate while the experimental group averaged 84 percent.

The rather startling relationship between physical fitness, regular fitness activities, and cerebral competence is not restricted to school-age youngsters. At the University of Illinois, physiologists Richard R. Powell and Richard H. Pohndorf compared mental tests of 26 older adult males who had participated in a running-type exercise regimen for three years with 22 men who exercised little or not at all during the same period. The "Culture Fair" intelligence test was administered to both groups; this test evaluates certain intelligence factors that often decrease as age increases in adults. The investigators found that the regular exercisers scored significantly higher than the nonexercisers. Similar results have been reported from studies of elderly patients tested for senility.

George Sheehan is fond of telling people that everyone should have some way of being an artist, that each of us was designed to do something best. "We become creative when we are in action," advises Sheehan, "then, we apply it later." The act of creating one's personal athlete can, itself, be the creative act. Kate Schmidt, winner of the bronze medal for the javelin throw in the 1976 Olympics, articulates this as she describes her growth as a competitor: "I love to see myself getting strong and improving my confidence." My conversations with hundreds of distance runners, swimmers, cyclists, and walkers support Dr. Sheehan's theory. Dick Traum, for example, is a New York management consultant; he is also one of the folk heroes among distance runners in America. Dick lost his right leg in an automobile accident several years ago. That kind of tragedy would have put most people on the sideline. Dick Traum demonstrates that he is very much in the game by running 26-mile marathons on an artificial limb. He described to me how his running not only keeps him fit and healthy but contributes to another important part of his life, his career. "First, I try to arrange my clients' problems in an orderly manner in my mind," said Dick. "Then, I go out for my daily run. After I'm out on the road for about an hour . . . zing! The results start to flash into my mind as though they were coming out of a computer." Dick also described how his concentration becomes enhanced to an incredible degree. "I often find that I can examine an object in my mind as though it were in three dimensions," he explained. "I can see a structure, such as a house or a client's plant, and I can turn it around, turn it upside down, look at it from all angles . . . it's fantastic." Sheehan experiences a "stream of consciousness," a cornucopia of ideas that becomes the basis for his writing. "I don't write my columns," he says. "I run them."

Psychologist Rollo May, in his book *The Courage to Create*, describes creativity as an encounter. The creative act ". . . may be sparked by the brilliant colors on the painter's palette or the inviting rough whiteness of the canvas." He likens the excitement and joy of that moment to a reenactment of the story of creation. Each of us who decides to resurrect our inner athlete, to restore ourselves as physical, mental, psychological, and spiritual beings, faces the creative encounter, an encounter with the soft, flabby, sedentary bench warmer that we may have been on the way to becoming. The colors shimmer on the palette and the canvas invites the man or woman who would pursue the ultimate adventure . . . growing to become the person that they were designed to be. How does one approach that challenge? One way is to go back to childhood, back to the time when we were still physical beings. There we will find our play.

6

The Athlete
Is a Sexual Being

Sexual pleasure, wisely used and not abused, may prove the stimulus and liberator of our finest and most exalted activities.

HAVELOCK ELLIS
Dance of Life

In 1978, an organization of law enforcement officers conducted a study of the effects of physical fitness programs on the lives and performance of policemen. As part of the survey, wives of policemen were queried as to their observations of the effects of physical fitness activities on their husbands. One of the most interesting responses was the wives' insistence that their newly fit police officer husbands had demonstrated a renewed enthusiasm for sexual activity. The surprising thing about this response was not that it occurred but that the wives knew why it had occurred.

One of the problems with trying to relate physical fitness to sexual performance — *sexual health* is a better term — is that most medical people are willing to support the premise "off the record" but are reluctant to come right out and say categorically that "if you exercise and become fit, your sex life will be improved." Of course, no guarantees can be made that exercise will have that result in any *specific* case. And such a relationship is all but impossible to prove even if it does seem to work.

The president of a large "Fortune 500" company has made fitness a corporate philosophy and attributes the success of his business to what he calls the "fitness edge." He articulates the relationship of fitness, longevity, and sexual health in a way that is meaningful to his employees and to the many audiences he addresses concerning health and fitness. "No one can *prove* that exercise prevents heart attacks, or causes us to live longer, or to maintain sexual vigor," he says. "But as we live our lives, there are certain things that have the ring of truth, which we believe in sufficiently to act on them, even if scientific method cannot establish proof." It is with such reasoning that so many older Americans find that, with fitness, they can stay active sexually.

Many people in our culture have grown up with major misconceptions about their sexuality and how aging affects it. On the one hand, there are those who believe that sexual activity contributes to aging; on the contrary, it can actually help us to retain our youth and vigor. Then, there are people who believe that sexuality is only for young folks. Again . . . not true. Our sexuality is one of the most exciting dimensions of life. It is a component of being a man or woman that makes one interesting and interested. It is the essence of the mystery and one of the beautiful things that make living worthwhile. When an individual loses that sense of his or her sexuality, you know they have lost their sense of life.

Sexual health can be likened in a sense to cardiovascular fitness. Earlier in this book it was pointed out that the heart is a muscle, and like any muscle it must be exercised or it degenerates. The same principle seems to apply to the psychophysiological sexual system. It is not uncommon for prisoners and others deprived of sexual contact for extended periods of time to lose interest in sexual activity. The sexual apparatus has to be used to remain healthy.

Frequently, we hear about such phenomena as "mid-life crisis" and "male menopause," and many people in their middle years are waiting apprehensively for something to happen to them sexually. Menopause in women, we know, is a specific physiological occurrence that takes place at about the fiftieth year. In addition to the fact that ovulation ceases, the ovaries produce considerably fewer estrogens. The physiological symptoms of menopause are largely understood today by women approaching or passing through this experience. What they should understand, however, is that the climacteric is not the signal that the male-female adventure is over. Neither should men entertain the fear that something specific is going to rob them of their sexuality.

The way to keep that adventure alive — for both men and women — is to work toward a physical and mental state that allows us to think of ourselves as sexually attractive and sexually functional people. Time and time again, when men and women in their middle years embark on physical fitness programs, the scenario usually goes something like this:

Sam is a fifty- (or forty- or sixty-) year-old accountant. He is thirty pounds overweight and has a body like a marshmallow. Recently he has had a few dizzy spells, he can't climb a flight of stairs without shortness of breath, his golf swing has gone to pot because he no longer has the body turn to get the club head back, and he's worried! Sam's sex life has degenerated to the point where he no longer feels that he is a really virile, sexually potent male. A couple of failures in bed have occurred, and Sam would really rather not risk any more embarrassments. He has suppressed his libido until even he is convinced it no longer exists. His mate is either dismayed at this turn of events or she is keeping pace with Sam . . . gradually retiring from the game.

But something happens to Sam. One of his clients has been running regularly for six or eight months, and one day Sam realizes that Lou has lost weight and looks years younger. "Lou, you look great," he observes. "Do you mean to tell me that exercise has done all this for you?" Lou affirms that, yes, he started jogging, gradually modified his eating and drinking habits, got more sleep, and that he feels as good as he looks.

Sam decides that exercise may be his last chance to rescue himself from himself. He checks with his doctor, then consults his local YMCA or perhaps he tries the programs in this book. Six months later he has lost twenty pounds, his jowls have disappeared, and he discusses running with Lou after every business meeting. Something else is beginning to happen to Sam. He doesn't feel like an old guy anymore. He finds that he can wear clothes better and even dares to try some of the new, more youthful styles. Sam's new self-image spills over into every dimension of his life. He feels more youthful, more confident, and more like a man again ... especially when he senses that women are beginning to notice him once more. Sam's new mental attitude is working in tandem with a healthier body. His exercise program has given him more stamina and vigor. His blood circulation has radically improved, resulting in rejuvenation of all of the organs in his body, including the sexual organs. It is likely that Sam's spouse will welcome his apparent rejuvenation and be a willing and enthusiastic sexual partner again.

Of course, the same kind of sexual degeneration and subsequent rejuvenation takes place among women when they adopt a fitness/growth lifestyle. Women are literally being reborn after finding a fitness activity that appeals to them. A whole new world opens up to them ... one they thought they had left forever. It's the world of exciting new clothing styles, smaller dress sizes, and the gleam of interest in a man's eye.

However, like most coins, even this one has another side. You can imagine the kind of problem that can develop when only one spouse — the husband or the wife — decides to get trim and fit and back in the game. A sexually active man or woman needs a sexually attractive partner. It is easy to see how a man and woman can grow farther apart rather than closer together if only one of them believes it is worthwhile to be physically and sexually attractive. I would be reluctant to make any specific suggestions as to how to get around that problem except to say — as I have done elsewhere in this book — that for a man and woman to embark on a fitness/growth program together is the great joy — and the true adventure.

7

How to Begin Your Training Program

Have you seen the fool that corrupted his own live
body? or the fool that corrupted her own live body?
For they do not conceal themselves, and cannot conceal themselves.

WALT WHITMAN
Children of Adam

We concluded in the first chapter that each of us is engaged in
a training program — training our minds and bodies either to
stay in the game as active, productive participants or to retire
to the bench as spectators.

The role we choose for ourselves depends on attitude, on pre-
conditioning. If we find ourselves among the spectators, the
job is to change. But before we can change lifestyles, we've got
to be able to change attitudes. In order to change attitudes it
is necessary to change ideologies or belief systems. The young
people of the 1980s are fortunate to be growing up during a
time when exercise and physical activity are on the upswing
in the United States. In a sense, it is *in* — among the young —
to be a jogger or a tennis player; it is *in* to be slim and athletic
looking; it is *in* not to smoke. Youngsters and young adults
with such an orientation will be slim and athletic and will be
living their lives in a manner designed to help them age well.
But many people in their middle years and older are more difficult to reach.

Recently, I spoke with Mike, a man in his middle seventies. Mike did hard physical labor all his working life and had always been hale and healthy, even though he was always a heavy smoker. Since retirement some ten years ago, he has done very little physical activity and no exercise. His belly protrudes now, and his smoking has begun to catch up with him; he pants audibly after any physical effort. Mike scorns exercise and refuses to believe that his smoking and his breathing problem are connected. "It's my age," he insists.

Tony is a newly retired bricklayer of 65. His job kept him fairly fit, but over the years he put on about 25 pounds of excess weight. "I wish I had gotten into something like this jogging when I was younger," he told me. Tony detests being out of shape. I advised him that it is never too late to begin and that even our local YMCA could put him on a safe program just right for his age and state of health. But Tony continues to hesitate. He is like the child at the edge of the swimming pool . . . afraid to take the plunge. All Tony's life he had been conditioned to believe that, when you got older, you were supposed to take it easy.

Eula Weaver is something else, altogether. Not long ago, I had the opportunity to write and produce *Coping with Life on the Run*, a film for TWA's inflight film program. The film dealt with health and physical fitness, and it gave me the opportunity to interview this wonderful, plucky lady. Almost ten years ago, at age 81, Eula Weaver experienced congestive heart failure. But Eula wasn't ready to leave the game. Here's how she tells it: "They told me I had just two chances. To go to bed, let them feed me with a spoon, carry me to the bath . . . or to get up and get out on the street." Eula describes how she lay there and thought it over. "When that little doctor came back," continued Eula, "I told him, 'I've got my mind made up.' Now I jog a mile a day and ride my bicycle up to twenty miles a day." Today, at almost ninety years of age Eula is still at it.

So, what we are really looking for is commitment ... the
kind of commitment that Eula Weaver proved could end up
being a rebirth. In order to embark on one's new training program, it is vital to understand what is going to be required and
why such a commitment should be made. It means a realistic
examination of ourselves. It can be a good idea to make a list
of all the things we do that are counterproductive, things like
smoking, overeating, eating large amounts of sweet or fatty
foods, abuse of alcohol, abuse of drugs, reliance on such medication as sleeping pills, tranquilizers, or analgesics. We may
fret and worry about our health — or about some other component of our lives. Such stress may cause tension and any
number of symptoms. Dr. Joan Ullyot, a nationally known preventive medicine specialist, author, and marathon runner, has
said, "It's shocking that half of our population is on Valium
when a run of two or three miles a day would do twice as
much good."

If we can see a picture of ourselves, of our lifestyle habits,
a picture that shows where we are headed, then our new training program will make sense. In April of 1977, I interviewed a
San Francisco businessman at Hopkinton, Massachusetts, just
before the Boston Marathon. He said, "Two years ago, I was
lying supine on the couch, like about ninety percent of the
males in the United States, watching the Super Bowl. I read
about the Bay to Breakers [a six-mile road race in San Fran-
cisco]. I weighed over two hundred pounds and I smoked and
I drank, but I decided to try it." He described how he ran
daily and worked his mileage up and the glorious feeling that
came with success. "I made it without stopping," he continued,
"and I said to my wife ... I'm going to run the Boston Marathon." The man I was talking to was about fifty years of age.
He was lean and suntanned and obviously in the full bloom of
health. We see here a classic case of sedentary living, self-
assessment, commitment, and rebirth into a joyful, rewarding
new lifestyle — one that features daily growth rather than
degeneration.

After commitment, immediate action is necessary. Most readers of this book should begin their course of action with a visit to their physician. Adults over 35, especially men who have led sedentary lives for many years, will want to have the doctor's OK before undertaking an exercise regimen. I suggest that you bring this book with you and tell him about your fitness and lifestyle goals. He will be delighted that you are ready to treat your new commitment to health, fitness, and personal growth as a team effort. Even professional sports teams and top athletes have a team physician, and your doctor can serve in that role. He will review the exercises and determine whether any of them might be beyond your capability or might have adverse effects because of specific illness or physical shortcomings.

Depending on your age and state of health, he may administer an ECG (electrocardiogram) to determine heart function or a stress ECG, which will tell him how your heart will respond to vigorous aerobic-type exercise. Today, physicians can tell a great deal about the state of the cardiovascular system simply by doing a blood chemistry test. In addition, the physician is often in the best position to ascertain which aerobic exercise might be best suited to your physiology. Older people, for example, may be better suited to walking or water exercise than to jogging or cycling, and the physician can offer advice on this. He will also insist on setting weight-loss goals.

Once you have your physician's go-ahead, your training program can commence. It is important to understand, at this point, that you are not simply going on a diet or undertaking a three-month exercise course. A diet implies changing one's eating habits temporarily to achieve a short-term weight-loss goal. It further implies that the dieter will return to his or her former eating habits at some time in the future, producing the familiar "yo-yo" effect of consecutive losses and gains in weight. Most exercise programs also imply some kind of short-lived Spartan regimen designed to achieve a kind of nebulous condition called "being in shape."

Staying in the game doesn't require doing anything drastic, today or tomorrow. Our training program is for the *big game*, and it means making small but permanent changes in the way we live our lives. The reward in our program will not be ending the "diet" or finishing the exercise program. The joy will be in the way we feel as we begin to clean up our act and get closer to the ideal "you" and "me." It will be the pride in being able to walk or jog another mile or being able to look in the mirror and admire what we see. And the special joy will be in knowing that — no matter what age we may be — we have added a growth component to our lives. We will know that we are a little stronger, slimmer, and more supple each day — that we are putting age aside.

The following chapters outline specific routines for men and women, as well as some simple techniques to determine one's cardiorespiratory fitness, muscle tone, and flexibility.

8

You've Got to Have Heart

The heart, consequently, is the beginning of life; the sun of the microcosm, even as the sun in his turn might well be designated the heart of the world; for it is the heart by whose virtue and pulse the blood is moved, perfected, made apt to nourish, and is preserved from corruption and coagulation; it is the household divinity which, discharging its function, nourishes, cherishes, quickens the whole body, and is indeed the foundation of life, the source of all action.

WILLIAM HARVEY, 1628

"The heart is a pump, a bloody pump. It sits somewhere in the upper middle of me. The statistics show that it is my number one enemy. I don't have to look out there — outside — for what is to get me; it's right here. A time bomb, two inches inside my chest, armed by fat and booze and smoke, pumping, ticking, clogging. Ready to stop." These words were written by Thaddeus Kostrubala, M.D. What strikes us about Dr. Kostrubala is that he's one of us. A guy frightened out of his tree by the very idea of having a heart attack. And you can believe that Thaddeus Kostrubala has thought about it. He continues: "When people die from a heart attack, they know it. There are those few seconds — ten or so, maybe even thirty — when, after the heart has stopped, they *know* it has stopped. I wonder what they do, what they think." It is impossible to read Dr. Kostrubala's words without reflecting on the condition of one's own heart, knowing as we do that heart disease

is the number one killer in America today. Such concern is
healthy and positive if it leads us to a plan of preventive maintenance for this most important organ. Cardiologist George
Sheehan points out that most of us have a seventy-year war-
ranty, but, if we want to live out that seventy years — and
more — and if we don't want to be in for repairs all the time,
we have to live our lives in such a way that undue deterioration
of the heart is avoided.

Heart disease is one of the maladies of modern man that can
be classified as both a disease of disuse and a disease of choice.
In any single individual, the causes of heart disease can vary
considerably. A number of contributing agents, known as coronary risk factors, may combine in various proportions to produce coronary heart diseases. These risk factors are generally
concluded to be the following:

Heredity. A history of heart disease in the family constitutes
a coronary risk factor. One who has had either or both parents
or a sister or brother succumb to a heart attack at an early age
must face the fact that they have probably inherited a coronary risk factor. This is one of the two risk factors over
which one has no control. The other follows.

Sex. Men — especially men under forty years of age — are
many times more likely to be heart attack victims than are
women of commensurate ages. It is only when a woman has
passed menopause that her susceptibility to heart disease increases. But statistically, even then she will remain behind her
husband in her proclivity toward heart disease. An interesting
outgrowth of the women's movement — and the increasing
proportion of women who smoke — is discernible in the change
in the proportions of men and women who experience heart attacks. As women enter the work force in greater numbers and
find themselves in more of the stress-associated managerial
and executive positions, they are finding themselves more and
more subject to stress-related ailments — like heart disease —
than before.

Smoking. Although most of us are aware of the cancer risks associated with smoking, there hasn't been as much public attention paid to the fact that smoking is a major coronary risk factor. Tobacco smoking is indisputably linked to diseases of the circulatory system, causing smokers to be roughly twice as susceptible as nonsmokers to heart attacks. Since fitness is a main focus of this book, it should be mentioned that Dr. Kenneth Cooper asserts that, "You simply can't smoke and be fit." Fortunately, we can do something about smoking and the other risk factors. They can be controlled.

Cholesterol. Cholesterol is one of the most controversial elements in the risk factor equation, because blood-serum cholesterol is determined by a number of influences that are not completely understood. It is known that the body manufactures cholesterol. It is also apparent that high cholesterol levels are related to the ingestion of large amounts of animal fats. High serum cholesterol levels clog blood vessels and contribute to coronary artery disease and strokes.

High Blood Pressure. High blood pressure is one of the major coronary risk factors. The reason it is so insidious is that high blood pressure is virtually symptomless. Only 4 persons out of 10 with high blood pressure even know that they have it. Blood pressure can be controlled by means of medication, diet, exercise, and relaxation techniques.

Overweight. Overweight or obesity as a coronary risk factor has obvious links to several of the others. Cholesterol levels and blood pressure are related to what and how much one eats, just as weight is. Being overweight causes the heart to work harder and saps one's energy. A person who has been overweight for most of his or her life may never know what it is like to feel really good.

Lack of Physical Activity. The lack of vigorous physical activity in one's daily routine has proven to be another common characteristic of the heart attack victim. People with jobs that keep them continually moving show a lower incidence of heart disease. A recent study of 17,000 Harvard graduates by Dr. Ralph S. Paffenbarger, Jr., confirmed that people who exercise regularly (accomplishing a 2000-calorie burn per week) have a marked decrease in the incidence of heart disease.

The heart is a muscle, and as with any other muscle, it must be regularly exercised and strengthened or else it begins to grow weaker. In this sense, heart disease is a disease of disuse. Sedentary living allows the heart muscle to slowly degenerate. At the same time, a sedentary lifestyle encourages the accumulation of weight in the form of body fat and elevated cholesterol levels, thus putting a constantly increasing load on a continually degenerating system.

Smoking and eating large quantities of fats and sugars are contributing factors confirming that coronary artery disease is also very much a disease of choice. It is easy to see how those ideas overlap. Behavioral scientists today understand that a characteristic like obesity indicates a lack of control, which influences other areas. For example, a person who eats too much is also likely to be inordinately fond of the wrong foods and is apt to be sedentary. The Center for the Application of Behavioral Science in St. Louis has set up a team to help people deal with such problems. Dr. David Munz, a psychologist who heads up the St. Louis center's Health Promotion and Positive Living Program, stresses physical exercise as the best way to help people to open up wide-sweeping lifestyle changes. "Once a person begins to achieve modest fitness goals," says Dr. Munz, "his self-image begins to change." Eventually he may not need to rely on the crutches offered by food, tobacco, drugs, or alcohol.

In terms of our training program, we are going to put cardiorespiratory fitness at the top of the list. Those of us who intend to stay in the game will have to have healthy hearts, and we are going to begin with exercise. Here's why. The overwhelming majority of reports on fitness from all over the world lend strong support to the inverse relationship between the amount of physical activity individuals indulge in and incidence of coronary heart disease. The conclusion is that a moderate level of physical activity throughout life is one of the factors that act to inhibit the degenerative characteristics of heart disease. Two internationally known researchers, Doctors Sam Fox and Paul Oglesby, report the following mechanisms by which physical activity may reduce the occurrence and severity of coronary heart disease:

1. *Increased coronary vascularization:* collateral circulation increased through exercise at and around the area of coronary restriction.

2. *Myocardial function:* enhancing myocardial efficiency. (The myocardium is the heart muscle [author's note].)

3. *Serum lipids:* lowering levels of serum cholesterol and serum triglycerides.

4. *Blood coagulation:* a favorable effect on blood clotting, stimulated by an increase in physical activity.

5. *Blood pressure:* reduction of blood pressure through exercise.

6. *Obesity:* physical activity combined with dieting is more effective in weight control than either program by itself.

7. *Psychic reactivity:* modify mental conflicts through physical activity, although still unproved.

One of the most exciting new discoveries about exercise concerns its effect on not only the *amount* but the *type* of cholesterol present in the blood. Serum cholesterol now is understood to be of two types: high density lipo-proteins (HDLs) and low density lipo-proteins (LDLs). The LDLs are the bad guys. Low density lipo-proteins are the sticky kind; they stick to each other and adhere to the walls of the blood vessels, forming the cholesterol "plaque" we often hear about. Exercise seems to increase the ratio of HDLs to LDLs, thus reducing the onset of arteriosclerosis and clogging of the coronary arteries. Chalk up another one for exercise!

So all of the research is conclusive: Exercise is good for our hearts. But, because of the kind of creatures we are, research seldom causes us to modify our habits. We are more likely to be influenced by the experiences of other people — people like us.

Acknowledging that it is impossible to state categorically that exercise has ever prevented a specific heart attack, I decided to go where the cause/effect relationship might be more demonstrable. Dr. Noel Nequin's cardiac rehabilitation program at Swedish Covenant Hospital in Chicago provided the kinds of case histories I was looking for.

Dr. Nequin, a pleasant, slightly built cardiologist, is a marathon runner himself and is one of the pioneer physicians who understood, almost instinctively, that exercise was the way to return cardiac victims to good health.

One of the most exciting interviews I experienced with Dr. Nequin's patients was with Dan, a tall, slim, strikingly handsome man about 35 years of age. A former pilot for one of America's leading airlines, Dan had experienced some disconcerting symptoms, and during one of his periodic physicals, it was determined that Dan had heart disease. He was, of course, immediately removed from flight status. "I felt like a vegetable," confided Dan. "All I did was sit around all day. I was really depressed. Then, I heard about this cardiac rehabilitation program at Swedish Covenant Hospital." Dan attended Dr. Nequin's 7 A.M. exercise classes five days a week even though it meant over 100 miles of driving each day.

A year later his ECG was normal. But it was to be another two years before Dan was allowed to climb aboard the flight deck of a commercial jet again as first pilot. "They really didn't want to return me to flight status," explained Dan. "It just wasn't done. But eventually they acknowledged that my physical and my stress tests checked out so much better than those of most of the other guys who were flying that it didn't make sense to keep me grounded any longer."

The day I spoke to Dan he held in his hands an official form from the F.A.A. examiners authorizing him to return to flight status and a letter from the airline for which he had worked inviting him to return for assignment. Dan was back in the game.

Another of Dr. Nequin's patients who stands out in my mind is Jim, a Chicago grocery executive. When Jim was 47 years of age, he experienced severe chest pain. He was overweight, sedentary, and disinclined to do anything physical. "I couldn't run across the street for a bus," Jim reported. Jim's physicians determined that he had severe blockage of all three major coronary arteries, and a triple by-pass was performed. Fortunately, Jim got some good advice. He was made to understand that the by-pass wasn't going to be the answer to his problem; whatever lifestyle factors had caused his artery blockages in the first place would cause the same thing to happen again unless the causative agents were removed. When Jim showed up at Dr. Nequin's office, he was fifty pounds overweight and, physically, just short of being a basket case. Jim was put on a walking program, then a jogging program, and finally a running regimen. Three years after he began the program, Jim entered the Mayor Daley Marathon — a full 26-mile marathon. The "Jim" I met was broad-shouldered, slim-waisted — an athlete, truly in the game for the first time. "My heart condition could have ended my life," Jim told me, "but instead it was the beginning. I've lost fifty pounds, I'm able to run a twenty-six-mile marathon, and at fifty years of age, I feel that I'm just beginning to really live."

9

Heart-Builder Programs for Fun and Fitness

The heart has its reasons which reason does not know.
PASCAL

Johnny Kelly is a well-known personage at the Boston Marathon. He is a white-haired, leprechaun-like man in his seventies who wears "Number 1" in the race each year. "This is my forty-sixth Boston," Johnny told me before the start of the 1977 Marathon. "Aside from winning once, I've finished in the first ten nineteen times. I've had a pretty good career, I guess." Johnny Kelly is no longer a contender for the winner's circle, but each year he goes out and wins it in a special and personal way, as so many other runners do. "If you finish a marathon, you're a winner," they say. "It used to be that there wasn't anyone over forty out here," remarked Kelly. "Now you see them in their forties, fifties, and sixties. As for me, I think it's wonderful. If I don't walk or run every day, I feel as though something has been stolen from me."

John Kelly is one of many marathoners in their seventies who seem to be able to go on forever. Such people measure their fitness in terms of the joy of being able to live life at the top of their powers, notwithstanding their chronological ages. How exciting — at any age — to have the ability to instruct the body to perform such a marvelous athletic feat and then to go out and do it. Shouldn't it be that way for each of us? Shouldn't every one of us be able to do our daily chores, handle crises and stress, and then have the energy, stamina, and enthusiasm to go for a run, a brisk round of tennis, a bracing bike ride, all without soreness or undue fatigue? George Blanda, who played professional football for the Oakland Raiders until he was 49, says that we don't want to be fit just so we can do our jobs better; we want to be fit so we can enjoy fun in life. The trim individual experiences his fitness in his zest for living. Exercise physiologists and other health professionals — the people who help us get fit — can measure our fitness in precise scientific terms. And they've devised ways by which we can test ourselves.

Dr. Kenneth Cooper, director of the Aerobics Fitness Center in Dallas and author of *Aerobics* and *The New Aerobics*, has developed the following tests (for men and women) that describe an individual's state of cardiorespiratory fitness or *aerobic capacity*. These tests are based on the distance one can walk or jog comfortably in 12 minutes. Dr. Cooper and his staff have determined that these tests compare with a treadmill measurement of oxygen consumption (aerobic capacity) with 90 percent accuracy.

First find an area — a track or roadway — where it is possible to determine distance covered. When you are ready to commence your test, make sure you have a stopwatch or a watch with a second hand or digital readout showing minutes and seconds. This way you can conduct your test for exactly 12 minutes, which is essential. Start out running or jogging. As soon as you begin to become winded, slow down to a walk until you recover, then run or jog again. Cover as much distance as you can without straining in 12 minutes. The following charts for men and women indicate your level of cardiorespiratory fitness. These tests are not recommended for persons in their post-retirement years, who should refer to Chapter 12, "A Total Program for the Later Years."

DR. COOPER'S 12-MINUTE TEST FOR MEN.
(Distance in miles covered in 12 minutes)

FITNESS CATEGORY	AGE			
	Under 30	*30–39*	*40–49*	*50+*
I. Very poor	<.1.0	<.95	<.85	<.80
II. Poor	1.0–1.24	.95–1.14	.85–1.04	.80– .99
III. Fair	1.25–1.49	1.15–1.39	1.05–1.29	1.0 –1.24
IV. Good	1.50–1.74	1.40–1.64	1.30–1.54	1.25–1.49
V. Excellent	1.75+	1.65+	1.55+	1.50+

< Means less than.

DR. COOPER'S 12-MINUTE TEST FOR WOMEN.
(Distance in miles covered in 12 minutes)

FITNESS CATEGORY	AGE			
	Under 30	*30–39*	*40–49*	*50+*
I. Very Poor	<.95	<.85	<.75	<.65
II. Poor	.95–1.14	.85–1.04	.75– .94	.65– .84
III. Fair	1.15–1.34	1.05–1.24	.95–1.14	.85–1.04
IV. Good	1.35–1.64	1.25–1.54	1.15–1.44	1.05–1.34
V. Excellent	1.65+	1.55+	1.45+	1.35+

The results of your 12-minute test will give you the harsh truth about where you stand in terms of cardiorespiratory fitness. Now you've got to decide what to do about it. Don't be discouraged if you didn't score well. Remember what this book is all about ... growth. If you don't rate well on the 12-minute test, you've got a great opportunity for improvement. It's important to remember, if you're severely out of shape, that it is due mostly to *inactivity* ... to your *old lifestyle* rather than to your age.

What can you do to make your heart-lung-circulatory system fit? You've got to find an aerobic-type exercise that suits you, one that will put sufficient stress on the cardiorespiratory system in a controlled manner. Such exercises include walking, jogging, cycling, and swimming. Dr. Kenneth Cooper's book *The New Aerobics* contains age-adjusted programs that translate the results of the aerobic tests described above into specific starter and aerobic fitness routines. These routines include all of the activities mentioned above. If you enjoy bike riding, make that your program. It will be far easier if it's something you like to do.

Before examining some of the more rigorous and structured cardiorespiratory activities, let's discuss the simplest one of all: walking. We hear a lot these days about the growth of jogging and running as sports and fitness activities. It is estimated that there are up to 25 million joggers today. But there are just as many walkers — maybe more. They are truly a "silent army." Maybe an invisible army would be a better description. They don't carry stopwatches or meet on Sundays for races, and they don't wear flashy warm-up suits. Neither have they adopted a uniform to distinguish them nor created for their pastime a mystique for cocktail party conversation. Yet ... they are out there. As with other fitness activities, many proponents begin at the advice of a physician. Some are post-cardiacs, some were obese, some had circulatory or even emotional problems. Most confirmed walkers do it because they love it.

How do you walk for fitness? Everyone knows how to walk. Right? Wrong. Even though all of us walk every day, the man or woman who decides to walk to fitness may encounter problems, or if not problems, he or she may not derive maximum advantage from walking without a bit of foreknowledge.

The first hurdle is to think of walking as fun. The automobile, the easy chair, and the desk have made many of us so used to sitting down that the idea of walking anywhere is rather shocking. In our culture, the only walking many of us do is from chair to chair. Once you rediscover walking, you will also rediscover a whole dimension of life that has been hidden from you. Older readers — especially those who are retired — can find a marvelous new adventure in walking, and it's free.

The first item for a new walker to consider is footwear. I highly recommend the shoes designed for jogging. They are light but sturdy. They have a good arch and excellent cushioning, and they are about the most comfortable shoes I've ever worn. They won't suffer drastically from the elements, either. Being primarily of nylon, plastic, and rubber construction, they are almost impervious to water damage. Your feet will get wet very easily, though, in these shoes. Socks can be a factor, as well. Many seasoned walkers like to wear a silk or thin cotton inner sock and a heavier cotton or wool outer sock. The inner sock reduces friction and helps to eliminate chafing and blisters. The outer sock provides cushioning, warmth, and the absorption of perspiration.

When you walk at a brisk pace you'll be surprised how warm your body will feel, even in cold weather; so you won't want to burden yourself with heavy clothing. Veteran walkers usually wear a couple of layers of light clothing: sweaters and a Windbreaker. Such items can be removed or added as needed and tied around the waist when they're not being worn. The secret of keeping warm during a walk or hike, without wearing heavy clothing, is to keep the hands, the feet, and the head warm. A warm hat is vital on a cold, windy day, because loss of body heat through the head is considerable — especially for the man with a bald spot. Gloves and warm socks will keep the extremities warm. A lined or windproof vest is great on windy or very cold days. Hot weather wear is a matter of common sense. Here, too, light cotton clothing is recommended. Make sure that walking shorts and upper wear are loose and comfortable to avoid chafing. Again, a hat can be good protection if you are going to be exposed to the sun.

Distance is another big consideration. Don't be too ambitious. Start slowly and build up your distances. If you walk until you are tired, you're going to find, to your dismay, that you still have to get home again. You've got the same distance to cover on your return trip. So take that into consideration when you plan your walk. You'll find that, as you begin to derive the benefits from walking — new vigor and pep, a trimmer body, a stimulating sense of fitness, and a zest for life — the meaning of distance will change. This is especially true if you vary your routine frequently so that each walk becomes a new experience. Walkers and joggers both experience this strange sense of the relevance of distance.

Is there such a thing as walking *technique* or *style?* Sure there is. Again, you may say to yourself, of course, I know how to walk; I do it every day of my life. What true walkers find out is that the walking style used in order to get from chair to chair doesn't always work so well out on the roads or foot trails. We find that many people who have been nonathletic or who carry more weight than they should tend to walk in a splay-footed manner — with the toes pointed out. Those who are working toward reestablishing the athlete within can learn something from watching amateur and professional athletes perform . . . even in such simple actions as walking or running. The baseball player digging for first base or the football half-back sprinting for the goal line will have his toes pointing in the direction in which his body is moving. When he walks, he does the same thing. The experienced walker knows that the most efficient, comfortable, and least tiring stride is one in which the toe reaches out in the direction toward which the walker is moving. A splay-footed walk causes the walker to waddle and to move from side to side rather than in a straight line. Even older walkers will find — after a short time — that we were really meant to walk straight.

Speed is another factor for the walker to consider. The neophyte will believe that walking at a slow leisurely pace is best. That's OK for a while — for the first couple of days; but as you straighten your stride out and begin to lengthen it a bit, you will want to step out and increase the pace. You should do this for two reasons: First, it's a matter of finding your own best stride. Surprisingly, most walkers find that the best pace is a fairly brisk one, because the body, like most mechanisms, functions best at a speed at which its own momentum becomes part of the rhythm. Three miles per hour seems to be the pace at which the body swings along at maximum efficiency covering the greatest distance with the least fatigue. The second reason for establishing an energetic pace becomes obvious when you recall why you are doing it in the first place. Your walking program is part of your training program; it's your form of aerobic exercise. If you can keep up a three-mile-an-hour pace, without straining, for a half hour, an hour, or more, you'll have no trouble staying in the game.

Just a word or two more on walking. Walking satisfies all of the definitions of play if it is done in a joyful, enthusiastic manner, and there are enough precedents for that. In his essay "Notes on Walking," Ralph Waldo Emerson describes walking as ". . . one of the secrets for dodging old age." Emerson did his best thinking as he strolled the hills, woodlands, and sea-shores of New England. "I think no pursuit has more breath of immortality in it," he advised his friends. Some of the world's most creative people are and have been walkers. Einstein strolled a country lane each morning as his mind soared across the reaches of time and space. Vladimir Nabokov claimed to have walked thousands of miles all over the world while, no doubt, visions of Lolita danced in his head. Plato was a walker, as were Charles Dickens, Christopher Morley, Thomas Mann, Robert Louis Stevenson, Henry David Thoreau, and Chief Justice Oliver Wendell Holmes. Harry Truman walked almost every day of his life because he believed it would help him to live longer; he lived to be 88.

You can walk to explore. You can walk to see the glorious sights of your home state, the nation, or a foreign land. You can walk to escape. You can walk to create. You can walk for the sheer fun of it — alone or with a companion. It's an excellent remedy for stress and a great heart builder.

Cycling is another form of aerobic exercise that can provide fun as well as fitness. The same guidelines apply to cycling in terms of pace and distance. The feeling that you should have when you do these exercises is one of slightly elevated respiration rate. You should be breathing at a more than normally rapid rate, but you should *not* be panting. If you can just about manage to carry on a conversation with a companion or sing a song if you are alone — without having to pause to catch your breath — you are exercising at exactly the correct rate. Exercise physiologists call this the "talk test." Sometimes a hill may cause you to become somewhat breathless, but you can recover by coasting down the other side. Clothing requirements are about the same as for walking, with less emphasis on footwear. Cycling provides all of the opportunities for touring and exploring that walking does but with considerably increased range. Bicycle tours of some of America's most scenic areas are now possible, and I know of several retired couples as well as family groups who have discovered a new world of excitement and adventure through this low-cost activity.

Swimming is another form of exercise that is rewarding in both fitness and fun. Everyone knows that swimming is an excellent conditioner, but not everyone has a pool or beach available on a year-round, daily basis. If you do, you can get a fine workout without the wear and tear imposed by the forces of gravity and friction that you experience in jogging, walking, or cycling. In the water, you are in a neutral density or weightless condition; all of the energy you expend is utilized to propel yourself through the water. This is an important consideration for someone with certain types of muscle or joint disease.

Approach swimming as an aerobic exercise, the same way as you do walking or cycling. Swim vigorously until a point of mild fatigue and slightly elevated respiration is achieved. Try to maintain this pace for at least 20 minutes three or four times a week. The rest of the time, just relax and enjoy the water.

It seems as though everyone wants to be a jogger these days. If the idea of jogging appeals to you, there is an incremental jogging program designed by the President's Council on Physical Fitness and Sports. This is a by-the-numbers, no-nonsense routine for those who are looking to achieve maximum fitness benefits, in the shortest amount of time, by using a programmatic approach. The program is set up in three parts, spanning 16 weeks. At the end of that 4-month period, you may discover that you would like to be a serious runner, maybe even do some road racing. You truly will have regenerated the athlete within you. Here's jogging program A:

Program A — Walking Program

Week	Daily Activity (*at least 3–4 times per week*)
1	Walk at a brisk pace for 5 minutes, or for a shorter time if you become uncomfortably tired. Walk slowly or rest for 3 minutes. Again, walk briskly for 8 minutes, or until you become uncomfortably tired.
2	Same as Week 1, but increase pace as soon as you can walk 5 minutes without soreness or fatigue.
3	Walk at a brisk pace for 8 minutes, or for a shorter time if you become uncomfortably tired. Walk slowly or rest for 3 minutes. Again, walk briskly for 8 minutes, or until you become uncomfortably tired.
4	Same as Week 3, but increase pace as soon as you can walk 8 minutes without soreness or fatigue.

When you have completed Week 4 of Program A, begin at Week 1 of Program B:

Program B — Walking-Jogging Program

Week	Daily Activity
1	Walk at a brisk pace for 10 minutes, or for a shorter time if you become uncomfortably tired. Walk slowly or rest for 3 minutes. Again walk briskly for 10 minutes or until you become tired.

2   Walk at a brisk pace for 15 minutes, or for a shorter time if you become uncomfortably tired. Walk slowly for 3 minutes.

3   Jog 20 seconds (50 yards). Walk 1 minute (100 yards). Repeat 12 times.

4   Jog 20 seconds (50 yards). Walk 1 minute (100 yards). Repeat 12 times.

When you have completed Week 4 of Program B, begin at Week 1 of Program C:

PROGRAM C — JOGGING PROGRAM

Week   *Daily Activity*

1   Jog 40 seconds (100 yards). Walk 1 minute (100 yards). Repeat 9 times.

2   Jog 1 minute (150 yards). Walk 1 minute (100 yards). Repeat 8 times.

3   Jog 2 minutes (300 yards). Walk 1 minute (100 yards). Repeat 6 times.

4   Jog 4 minutes (600 yards). Walk 1 minute (100 yards). Repeat 4 times.

5   Jog 6 minutes (900 yards). Walk 1 minute (100 yards). Repeat 3 times.

6   Jog 8 minutes (1200 yards). Walk 2 minutes (200 yards). Repeat 2 times.

7   Jog 10 minutes (1500 yards). Walk 2 minutes (200 yards). Repeat 2 times.

8   Jog 12 minutes (1700 yards). Walk 2 minutes (200 yards). Repeat 2 times.

Remember that it is important to warm-up and cool-down before and after all of the aerobics activities outlined in this chapter. (Refer to Chapter 10, "Get Loose, Stay Loose," for the recommended warm-up and cool-down exercises.)

Exercise physiologists have determined that the best and fastest way to develop cardiorespiratory fitness is to elevate the heart rate, through exercise, to a specific level and maintain it at that level for 20 minutes or more at least three times per week, preferably on alternate days. When this is done, a "training effect" takes place, which means that the heart, lungs, and circulatory system are improving their efficiency. It means that your "heart-builder" program is working. The level to which you should elevate your heart rate during aerobic-type exercise is called your "target zone." It can be determined quite accurately during an electrocardiogram taken when the body is being stressed. This is known as an *exercise* ECG. The target zone resulting from such a test tells you the minimum heart rate necessary for you to experience a training effect and the maximum rate that you should allow your heart to achieve.

How does one know what his or her target zone is? It is based on exercising at a specified percentage of an individual's *maximum achievable heart rate*, and that figure is a function of one's age. Assuming that you have not had an exercise ECG, you can determine your appropriate maximum achievable heart rate by subtracting your age from the number 220. For example, a fifty-year-old man or woman has a theoretical maximum heart rate of 170 beats per minute.

Conditioning is best achieved when you're exercising at a pace that elevates the heart rate to the target zone that lies between 70 and 80 percent of your maximum achievable heart rate. The heart rate should not be allowed to exceed 80 percent of the maximum rate. The following chart gives sample target zones for various age groups.

PERCENTAGE OF MAXIMUM HEART RATE

Age	70 Percent	80 Percent	100 Percent
18–29	142–134	162–153	203–191
30–39	133–127	152–145	190–181
40–49	126–120	144–137	180–171
50–59	119–113	136–129	170–161
60–69	112–106	128–121	160–151
70–79	105– 99	120–113	150–141

In each pair of figures in the chart, the highest heart rate relates to the lowest age and the lower heart rate is for the older end of the age group. To find your specific target zone or exercise range, subtract your age from 220, take 70 percent of that number as the low end of your target zone; take 80 percent of the same number as the high end of your target zone. Check your results against the chart for accuracy.

In order to use this information, you will have to be able to read your pulse, which beats at the same rate as your heart. Here's how to do it: Place the finger tips of one hand on the artery located in the top, inside of the wrist of your other hand. If you have difficulty locating a pulse beat there, you will find a strong beat at either of the two carotid arteries in the neck. Simply place your thumb on your chin and reach around with your index finger until you feel the large muscle running down your neck from behind your ear. Right in front of this muscle — between the muscle and your windpipe — you will find a strong pulse. Using either of these methods, count your pulse for 6 seconds and multiply the result by 10. This will tell you your heart rate in beats per minute. If you are jogging, cycling, swimming, or skipping rope, your exercise pulse will tell you if you are in your target zone. If you are below the target zone, pick up the pace a bit; if your heart rate exceeds the target zone, slow down immediately. Walkers will find that their heart rates may never quite make it into the target zone. If you are a walker, don't allow that to worry you. Walking is usually sustained for a much longer period of time than the more rigorous aerobic exercises. Thus, the aerobic benefits are linked more closely to the *duration* of the activity than to the intensity.

Once you have become adept at reading your pulse, another revealing technique for measuring fitness becomes available to you. It's your *resting pulse rate*. Initially your heart rate, when you are *not* exercising, won't tell you very much. It can vary anywhere from the 70s to the 90s for most adults. Highly trained athletes have heart rates down as low as 40 beats per

minute. Once you have your aerobic fitness program under
way, you can monitor your progress in the following manner:
Every morning when you awaken, measure your pulse rate and
write it down. Do this before you get up, while your body is
still relaxed and at rest. Your resting heart rate should be
fairly consistent from day to day if you measure it at the
same time and under the same conditions. But after you have
been exercising for a couple of weeks, something will begin
to happen. You'll find that your resting heart rate is going
down. It may be 70 beats per minute when you start your
program and be down to 67 beats two months later. That
means that your cardiorespiratory fitness has improved. It
means that your "heart-builder" program has produced results. Your heart muscle is stronger. Your heart pumps more
blood than before with each beat, so it doesn't have to work
so hard at rest. Consequently, it can beat more slowly and
still accomplish the same amount of work. When you see that
happening — and you will — you'll know that you are *growing* in health and fitness and that's just the opposite of what
aging was supposed to do to you.

10

Get Loose, Stay Loose

Consider the planets swinging around the sun without
effort... Consider yourself a part of the cosmic motion. What would it be like if you were connected to
the swing of the planets?

GEORGE LEONARD
The Ultimate Athlete

One physical shortcoming almost always associated with aging
is the loss of flexibility, loss of the full range of body motion.
Older people speak of their "aching muscles and creaking
joints," and eventually we come to believe that it is all part
of the aging process. Not so! Not for those who intend to stay
in the game. Loss of body motion and many diseases of the
muscles and joints are maladies that we passively inflict on
ourselves by *allowing* our muscles to degenerate and our joints
to stiffen.

One of the most pervasive ailments of our time is low back
pain. Almost every family in America has had firsthand experience with low back disorders. Back pain is a prime example
of how stress and tension attack the deconditioned individual.
The President's Council on Physical Fitness and Sports and
its consultant on low back disabilities, orthopedist Hans Kraus,
emphasize that maladies of the low back are, for the most part,
preventable. The type of preventive and remedial exercise that
Dr. Kraus prescribes for his patients is primarily designed to
promote flexibility.

Arthritis, bursitis, and tendinitis are other ailments linked
to physical activity. An apparent contradiction seems to appear here. Many people experience pain associated with these
diseases when they attempt exercise or a sport, because the
body may have been ravished for years by sedentary living.
The muscles and joints simply aren't prepared for vigorous activities. Dramatic examples of this frequently show up at the
company picnic or the father-son softball game. But it is becoming more evident every day that individuals who exercise
regularly, who stay with their sport, who maintain their muscle
tone and flexibility are less susceptible to these ailments.

It isn't hard to understand why flexibility is so important if
we examine just what happens to muscles and joints as time
passes. Muscles that are used frequently become stronger,
tighter, and less supple than muscles that aren't used often.
Think about walking, for example. Almost everyone walks —
even if it's only from chair to chair. When we walk we use the
muscles in the backs of the legs (the calf muscle and the hamstring muscle in the back of the thighs) and muscles in the
buttocks and lower back. Consequently, these muscles become
stronger and tighter than the "front muscles" (the shin muscles
and the quadricep muscles in the front of the thighs and abdominal muscles). So, we have a situation with short, tight
muscles affecting the spine in the back and loose, slack muscles failing to support the spine in the front. It's like the mast
of a sailboat with only one guy wire. The low back begins to
develop an exaggerated curve as the belly protrudes. This condition is called "lordosis" and is a postural problem that afflicts
many Americans as they become less physically active and
grow older. Anyone with tight back muscles and loose, flabby
abdominal muscles is extremely vulnerable to a low back dis-
order. All it takes is a bit of strain from lifting, or from entering
an automobile, or it may even be a stressful incident in daily
life and wham . . . a low back spasm. When we speak of getting
"in shape," what we are talking about is acquiring flexibility

in our tight muscles and strength for our loose, slack muscles.

The joints, themselves, are subject to stiffening if they are not exercised regularly and properly. When you do the stretching exercises found in this chapter, you will be gently stretching the ligaments, tough bands of tissue that bind the joints together. People of all ages are amazed at the amount of flexibility that can be attained when they do these exercises on a regular basis. With increased flexibility comes the ability to play a sport better with less likelihood of injury, less soreness after a sports or exercise session, reduced risk of low back disability, and best of all, a body that moves and feels like a young body, regardless of age.

How to Stretch. When you begin the flexibility exercises in this chapter, the watchword is *moderation.* Stretching is supposed to feel good. If it hurts, you're stretching past your limits. Don't bounce when you stretch. This causes a reflex shortening of the muscle that is counterproductive. Hold each stretch for about 10 seconds and repeat 2 or 3 times unless otherwise specified.

Warm Up . . . Cool Down. Begin every exercise session with a warm-up period, even your aerobic program. The warm-up is meant to gradually increase your respiration rate and body temperature as well as to stretch ligaments and connective tissue. The cool-down period is meant to accomplish the reverse. You can cool down from your aerobic program by walking for 5 to 10 minutes with some of the following mild stretching exercises. The first seven of the following flexibility exercises can be your regular warm-up before all of your workouts.

1. Head Circles

Starting Position:
Stand erect, feet shoulder-width
apart, hands at sides.

Action:
Allow your head to tilt forward
until chin touches chest. Rotate
your head in a slow circle to the
right until you return to the starting position. Repeat this action
to the left.
Repeat 2 to 3 times, each side.

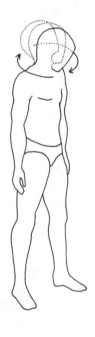

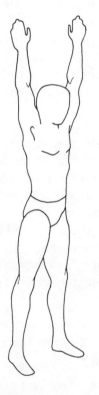

2. Standing Reach

Starting Position:
Stand erect, feet shoulder-width
apart and arms extended over
your head.

Action:
Stretch as high as possible, keep-
ing heels on the floor.
Hold for 15 to 30 counts.

3. Flexed-Leg Back Stretch

Starting Position:
Stand erect, feet shoulder-width apart, arms at your sides.

Action:
Slowly bend over, touching the floor between your feet. Keep your knees flexed. Hold for 15 to 30 counts. If at first you can't reach the floor, touch the tops of your shoes.
Repeat 2 to 3 times.

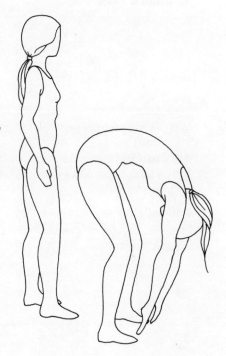

4. Alternate Knee Pull

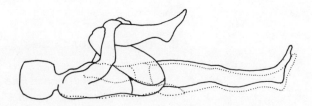

Starting Position:
Lie on your back, feet extended, hands at your sides.

Action:
Pull one leg to your chest, grasp with both arms and hold for a 5 count. Repeat with the opposite leg.
Repeat 7 to 10 times with each leg.

5. Double Knee Pull

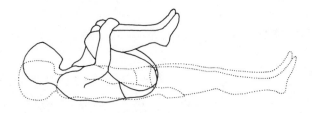

Starting Position:
Lie on your back, feet extended, hands at your sides.

Action:
Pull both legs to your chest, lock arms around legs, and pull your buttocks slightly off the floor. Hold for 20 to 40 counts.
Repeat 7 to 10 times.

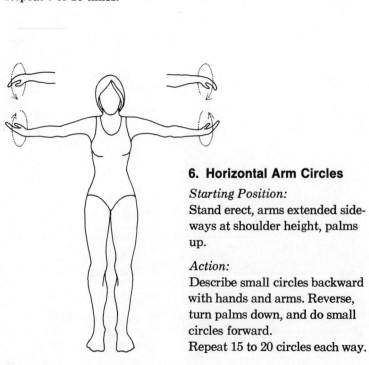

6. Horizontal Arm Circles

Starting Position:
Stand erect, arms extended sideways at shoulder height, palms up.

Action:
Describe small circles backward with hands and arms. Reverse, turn palms down, and do small circles forward.
Repeat 15 to 20 circles each way.

7. Giant Arm Circles

Starting Position:
Stand erect, feet shoulder-width apart, arms at your sides.

Action:
Bring arms upward and sideways, crossing over head, completing a full arc in front of your body. Suggested repetitions: Repeat 10 times, an equal number in each direction.

8. Back Leg Swing

Starting Position:
Stand erect behind a chair, with feet together and hands on the chair for support.

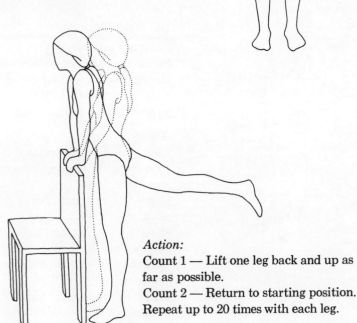

Action:
Count 1 — Lift one leg back and up as far as possible.
Count 2 — Return to starting position.
Repeat up to 20 times with each leg.

9. Side-Lying Leg Lifts

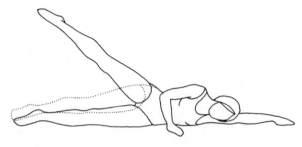

Starting Position:
Lie on your right side, with your leg extended.

Action:
Count 1 — Raise your left leg as high as possible.
Count 2 — Lower to starting position.
Repeat on opposite side, 10 to 15 times each side.

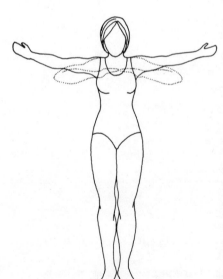

10. Wing Stretches

Starting Position:
Stand erect with your elbows at shoulder height and your arms bent so that the finger tips of your two hands are touching.

Action:
Count 1 — Pull elbows back as far as possible, keeping them at shoulder height.
Count 2 — Return to starting position.
Count 3 — Swing arms outward, maintaining shoulder height, until they are straight out from shoulders.
Count 4 — Return to starting position.
Repeat 10 to 20 times.

11. The Cobra

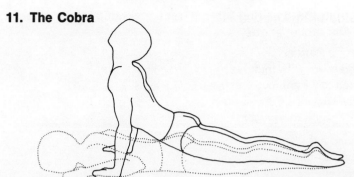

Starting Position:
Lie flat on the floor, face down, with your legs and feet extended.

Action:
Count 1 — Lift your head and slowly roll it backward. Hold for about 3 seconds.
Count 2 — Return to starting position.

12. Achilles Stretch (recommended for joggers and racket sports)

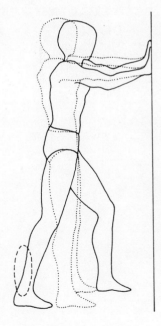

Starting Position:
Stand at arms' length from the wall, with both palms pressed against the wall.

Action:
Count 1 — Move one leg forward one half step, move the opposite leg back one half step.
Count 2 — With the heel of the rear leg held to the floor, lean toward the wall, stretching your calf muscle and Achilles' tendon.
Count 3 — Hold for 5 to 10 counts.
Repeat 3 to 6 times, each leg.

13. Upright Hamstring Stretch (recommended for joggers and racket sports)

Starting Position:
Stand erect, with right leg extended and right foot supported by the back of a chair or other object of suitable height.

Action:
Count 1 — Slide your hands down your leg to your right ankle.
Count 2 — Bend forward, bring your head as close to the right knee as possible. (Don't worry if, at first, you find this difficult.)
Count 3 — Hold for 10 to 15 counts.
Count 4 — Return to starting position.
Repeat 3 to 5 times with each leg.

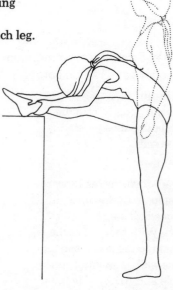

14. Legover (great for joggers, good for low back)

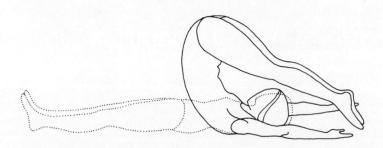

Starting Position:
Lie on the floor, with your arms extended over your head.

Action:
Count 1 — Carefully and slowly bring your legs over your head.
Count 2 — Straighten your legs and bring your toes as close to the floor as possible.
Count 3 — Hold for 5 counts. (If it is painful, relax the tension by bending your knees slightly.)
Count 4 — Return to the starting position.

It is recommended that you do these stretching and flexibility exercises at least three times a week, but many people find that because they feel so good they do them every day. If you want to prevent low back problems or if you have suffered from low back pain, exercises 3, 4, 5, 9, 13, and 14, together with the abdominal exercises in the next chapter, will provide protection. If you do have a back problem, check with your physician before doing these or any other exercises.

Anyone who has been sedentary for many years might be well advised to begin his or her training program here, with flexibility. Get your body used to moving again. Many of these exercises are conditioners as well as stretching activities, so muscle tone will begin to improve right away. Older readers, especially, will find that, once flexibility begins to be restored, a whole new rebirth of the body will take place.

11

Strength, for Durability

Fatigue makes cowards of us all.
VINCENT T. LOMBARDI

A physician friend of mine was attempting to explain the basic elements of fitness to a woman patient in her forties. He mentioned strength as a basic component of fitness along with flexibility and cardiorespiratory endurance. "Strength," she scoffed. "Why would I need strength? I can use a canopener and carry a laundry basket when I have to. Why should I do exercises to increase my strength?" Strength is surely a misunderstood quality among both men and women. It is an attribute that they expect to lose as they age, and that fact is not one of very great concern to most people.

But strength is essential. Anyone who expects to be a participant throughout life, who looks forward to maintaining a functional body into the later years, must develop and maintain strength. Together with flexibility, it is the quality that makes movement possible, and sport and everyday living a joy. Don't think of strength as something only football players and wrestlers need. Neither should you associate it with large bulging muscles. Boys, girls, men, and women of all ages need strong bodies.

If I were to ask you to create a mental image of an "old person" you might, unfortunately, visualize a person who is tottering, stooped over, almost helpless. You would be picturing someone who had lost his or her physical strength and flexibility. It's a picture you would do well to erase from your mind because, through your training program, you are going to avoid that eventuality. Studies show that human beings do, indeed, lose muscle strength as they age. But these studies fail to tell us that they are based on deterioration that takes place without physical training. In other words, a well-trained individual like Walter Stack, who, at 75 years of age, swims San Francisco Bay every morning after jogging 10 miles, has far greater muscle strength than many a deconditioned former athlete thirty years his junior. As I have emphasized continually in this book, it is improvement that we are concerned with, being a little stronger today than yesterday. That's growth, and it's the opposite of aging.

There are good reasons to develop strength and to keep it up. The obvious one is that being strong enables us to do our daily chores, to be productive, and then, at the appropriate times, to do the active things that are fun to do. It's so marvelous for a parent or a grandparent to be able to go hiking or backpacking with the children of the family or to join them in a game of volleyball or tennis. To do these things one must maintain strength, flexibility, and endurance.

A less obvious reason to be strong concerns the durability of the body itself. As the years pass, the body is engaged in a never-ending battle against gravity. The muscular-skeletal system either succumbs to the relentless pull of our planet or it steels itself to fight back. The person who neglects to preserve muscular-skeletal strength is going to find himself or herself "bowed by the years," as the poets say. Women are especially vulnerable to the gradual collapse of the body and its organs as they grow older. Many women have avoided exercise, especially those exercises that strengthen the abdominal muscles. Additionally, it is the rare person who has not gone on an occasional "crash diet." Each of these diets, if not accompanied by appropriate exercise, results in loss of muscle tissue as well as fat. Eventually, the muscles deteriorate to a point at which they can no longer support the organs of the body. As the body begins to sag — internally and externally — circulation is impaired and degenerative diseases of all kinds occur. It is heartbreaking to see such great numbers of middle-aged men and women entering the degenerative sequences that begin with physical deconditioning.

The strength exercises shown here are basic conditioning exercises designed to include all of the large muscle groups. These exercises will help the average man or woman achieve and maintain a desirable level of muscular-skeletal strength. Older readers can refer to the next chapter, "A Total Program for the Later Years." Other readers may wish to advance to more rigorous programs. Local Ys can provide such programs, and there are several excellent fitness books available in bookstores that include weight training and strength programs for specific sports. The following exercises are recommended by the President's Council on Physical Fitness and Sports. Be sure to do your warm-up and stretching exercises before these conditioners.

1. Head and Shoulder Curl (beginner)

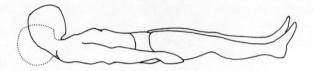

Starting Position:
Lie on your back, legs straight, arms at your sides.

Action:
Count 1 — Curl your head and shoulders off the floor. Hold this position for 5 counts.
Count 2 — Return to starting position.
Repeat: 10 to 15 times.

1a. Sit-up, Arms Crossed (intermediate)

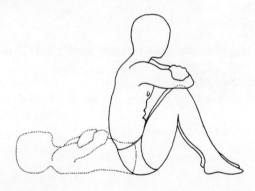

Starting Position:
Lie on your back, arms crossed on your chest, hands grasping opposite shoulders, knees bent with your heels close to your buttocks.

Action:
Count 1 — Curl up to a sitting position.
Count 2 — Curl down to the starting position.
Repeat: 10 to 15 times.

1b. Sit-up, Fingers Interlaced (advanced)

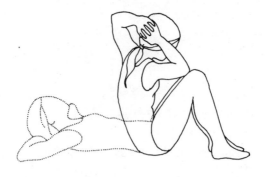

Starting Position:

Lie on your back with your knees bent, and your heels close to your buttocks, fingers of both hands interlaced behind your head. You may find it necessary to anchor your feet under a chair or other heavy object.

Action:

Count 1 — Curl up to a sitting position and touch right elbow to left knee.

Count 2 — Curl down to a sitting position.

Count 3 — Curl up to sitting position and touch left elbow to right knee.

Count 4 — Curl down to the starting position.

2. Knee Pushup (beginner)

When doing these exercises, it is important to keep the back straight. Start with the knee pushups and continue for several weeks until your stomach muscles are strong enough to keep your back straight. Then try the intermediate pushups.

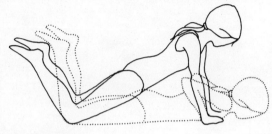

Starting Position:
Lie prone, hands alongside your shoulders, fingers pointing forward.

Action:
Count 1 — Straighten arms, keeping back straight.
Count 2 — Return to the starting position.
Repeat: 5 to 10 times.

2a. Pushup (intermediate)

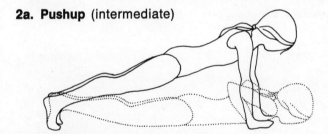

Starting Position:
Lie prone, hands outside your shoulders, fingers pointing forward, feet on the floor.

Action:
Count 1 — Straighten your arms, keeping your back straight.
Count 2 — Return to the starting position.
Repeat: 10 to 20 times.

2b. Chair Pushups (advanced)

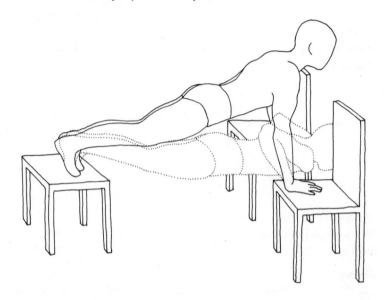

Starting Position:
Support your body on your hands on the edges of two chairs placed slightly outside of shoulders, fingers pointing forward. Your body should be straight, with your feet resting on another chair.

Action:
Count 1 — Lower your body as far as possible, bending your elbows.
Count 2 — Push your body up to the starting position.
Repeat: 5 to 10 times.

3. Sitting Single Leg Raises

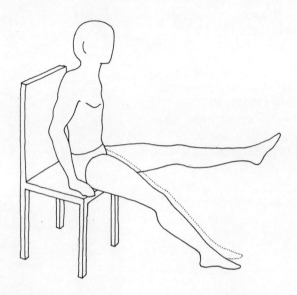

Starting Position:
Sit erect, hands on the sides of your chair seat for balance, legs extended at an angle to the floor.

Action:
Count 1 — Raise your left leg waist-high.
Count 2 — Return to the starting position.
Repeat an equal number of times with the opposite leg.
Repeat: 10 to 15 times.

4. Quarter Knee Bends

Starting Position:
Stand erect, hands on hips, feet comfortably spaced.

Action:
Count 1 — Bend your knees to about a 45-degree angle, keeping your heels on the floor.
Count 2 — Return to the starting position.
Repeat: 15 to 20 times.

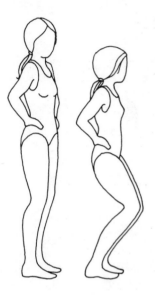

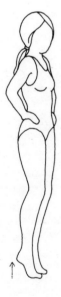

5. Heel Raises

Starting Position:
Stand erect, hands on hips, feet together.

Action:
Count 1 — Rise on your toes.
Count 2 — Return to the starting position.
Repeat: 20 times.

12

A Total Program
for the Later Years

The greater part of progress is the desire to progress.
SENECA (the younger)
Epistulae ad Lucilium

For purposes of definition, we'll define the "later years" as the post-retirement period in one's life. For many Americans this is a crucial time. For most of us the retirement years represent the rewards of the working years. It is the time of life when the pressures and stresses of job, career, or profession are supposed to disappear. Similarly, family responsibilities ease up as one's children pursue their own careers and family involvements. Retirement is the time when we imagine we will do all of the things we have dreamed of doing. It may mean travel or playing golf every day or fishing. Whatever our individual dream is, it lies out there shimmering in the future — in the golden years ahead.

Pensions, retirement programs, and social security provide many citizens with the financial resources to sustain themselves in some fashion after leaving the job. So, perhaps, if inflation hasn't chewed away at the dollar too drastically, some of the dreams of a lifetime may be possible of attainment after retirement . . . provided one is up to it physically and mentally. One of the great tragedies of our time is the large number of men and women struck down by diseases of disuse, diseases of choice as they approach and enter the later years. These are people who will never reach the golden years, never realize the dream. Many people who do reach retirement find that they are no longer able to *live* the dream. They are obese or afflicted with cardiovascular disease or high blood pressure or stiffness of the muscles and joints or any number of diseases associated with aging that we have called diseases of choice and diseases caused by disuse of the body. We know that it doesn't have to be that way, that this can be one of the best parts of the game. It's no time to be benched. This is when we need the physical activity of our training program more than ever.

While researching this chapter, I had an opportunity to observe fitness programs all over the United States, many of them being used by older people, people in their later years. I was looking for a routine that would deliver the maximum benefits in all components of fitness that are important to this age group. The program would have to restore full range of body motion; it would have to develop muscle tone, agility, and balance; it would have to rejuvenate the cardiovascular system — all without placing excess stress on the body or causing pain or discomfort. The *total program for the later years* that I am presenting here is derived from two programs that I observed and that satisfy the criteria outlined above. The exercises are selected from routines developed by the President's Council on Physical Fitness and Sports and by the Health Promotion Team at St. Louis University Medical Center. You should check this program with your physician, as I suggested earlier. I am sure he will encourage you to begin this routine. Even the most conservative doctor will agree that a "reasonable" amount of exercise is beneficial. This program starts you off with a very mild regimen, but it will take you to a remarkable level of fitness if you stay with it.

THREE LEVELS . . . STARTER TO ADVANCED

The exercises in this program are presented at three levels: starter, intermediate, and after about 6 to 9 weeks, the advanced. These levels of activity are designed to take the sedentary reader up to his or her desired goal of fitness. The reader who performs the routine three or four times a week will be strengthening and stretching all major muscle groups and, most important, improving the performance of the cardiovascular system. I suppose that everyone knows that the major problem with exercise programs is getting people to stick to them. Here are two tips that will help you to make your training program a permanent fixture in your life. First of all, find some time during the day — about half an hour — which will be your exercise time. If you find that doing the following program four times a week is the right frequency for you, go for a zesty 30-minute walk or bike ride on the alternate days. This will reinforce the idea that your exercise time is to be set aside for some kind of conditioning activity and that these activities can be fun. The second piece of advice I can offer that will help to make your exercise program permanent is to take it slow and easy. Many people of all ages have been detoured from their exercise activities because they overdid them; consequently, their first experience with exercise was painful and exhausting. If you move along slowly and easily with your program, you'll begin to feel stronger, looser, and more vigorous, and you'll enjoy these feelings. You'll know that this is the way you are supposed to feel. Your exercise session will become one of the most important parts of your day.

It is necessary that you follow the exercise plan exactly as it is laid out, even if it seems very easy in the beginning. If an exercise calls for only two or three repetitions, don't do any more. When you reach the advanced-level program, you will have the option to add repetitions and otherwise adjust the program to your personal requirements. By that time, you will have a better feel as to how your body is responding to the demands of various exercises. Earlier in this book I have emphasized the importance of warming up and cooling down as part of your workout. This routine has incorporated a warm-up and a cool-down, so the exercises should be performed in the sequence indicated.

How to Begin the Program

Once you begin your routine, you should try to work your way through it at a steady comfortable pace without stopping to rest too frequently. If you begin to feel overtaxed or dizzy, by all means slow down or stop and rest; but once you find your pace you will be able to maintain it and improve upon it. As your fitness improves and you find that you can do the exercises at a faster clip, be careful that you don't substitute speed for correct performance. At that point you are probably ready to move up to the next level.

For the first week or so, limit the number of repetitions or the duration of each exercise to the smallest number given. Even this may be too strenuous for you. If so, reduce the pace even more and don't increase it for another week or until you feel that you are ready. After you have completed the first week, or when you know that you are ready, increase the number of repetitions for each exercise by one repetition. For the next three to four weeks, gradually increase the number of repeats for each exercise, or the duration when applicable, until you are ready to move up to the intermediate level.

Proceed with the intermediate level the same way as outlined for the starter level. Work out at the intermediate level for about 3 to 5 weeks, or longer if necessary, once again increasing repeats and duration very gradually.

Eventually, you will be able to tackle the advanced level and you are going to enjoy a real sense of accomplishment. Continue just as you have been doing — increasing your level of activity at a slow, steady pace. When you can do the advanced level workout for three consecutive days without undue fatigue, you will have achieved a very satisfactory level of fitness. You'll be delighted at how good you feel, how your range of body motion has increased. You'll be thrilled at your new sense of strength and vigor. At this point, you can (1) continue with the exercises in this chapter, gradually increasing the number of repeats and the distances walked and jogged. You can also spend more time at sports and recreational activities that require physical effort, such as cycling, swimming, hiking, etc. (2) You may wish to advance to one of the more rigorous programs described in earlier chapters. (3) You can become a serious jogger or cyclist and graduate into competition. (4) You may become a dedicated athlete and compete in such programs as the Master Program run by the Amateur Athletic Union (A.A.U.) or the Senior Olympics.

Your Total Program

Each of the following exercises is illustrated where necessary and figures appear indicating the number of repeats or the duration of the exercise. Always start out using the lower number and gradually work up to the higher figures.

1. Warm-up Walk

Starter — 2 minutes
Intermediate — 3 minutes

2. Alternate Walk-Jog

Advanced level only — Walk 50 steps then jog 50 steps — 3 minutes
(Tips on jogging and walking are provided in the "Heart-Builder" chapter.)

3. Salute to the Sun

Starter — 2 to 10 times
Intermediate — 10 times
Advanced — 10 times

Position:
Stand erect with feet shoulder-width apart.

Count 1. Extend your arms overhead, reaching as high as possible and arching your back.
Count 2. Bend forward at the waist, stretching in a gentle attempt to touch finger tips to your toes. Flex your knees slightly while bending forward.
Count 3. Back to starting position.

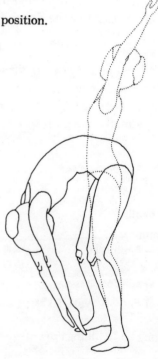

4. Shoulder Shrug

All levels — 3 to 5 times

Position:
Stand erect with hands at sides.
Count 1. Raise both shoulders
upward.
Count 2. Allow your shoulders
to drop back to their normal
position.

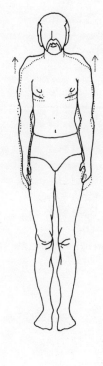

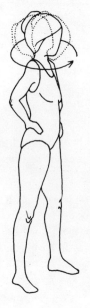

5. Neck Stretcher

Starter — 2 to 10 times each way
Intermediate — 10 times each way
Advanced — 10 times each way

Position:
Stand erect with hands on hips,
feet shoulder-width apart.

Count 1. Close your eyes and
slowly rotate your head in a full
circle from left to right.
Count 2. Slowly rotate your head
in the opposite direction.

6. Side Stretch

Starter — 2 to 5 times
Intermediate — 5 to 10 times
Advanced — 10 times

Position:
Stand with feet shoulder-width apart and hands extended overhead, finger tips touching.

Count 1. Bend your torso slowly to the left, as far as possible. Keep the hands together and the arms straight.
Count 2. Return to the starting position.
Counts 3 and 4. Repeat to the right.

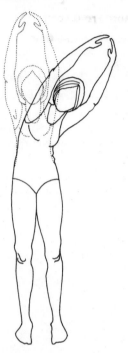

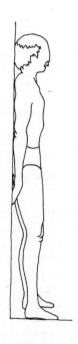

7. Back Straightener

Starter — 2 to 5 times
Intermediate — 5 times
Advanced — 5 times

Position:
Stand with your heels about 3 inches from wall, back pressed against it and head straight.

Count 1. Draw in your stomach by tightening the abdominal muscles and press the small of your back tight against the wall. Hold for 6 seconds.
Count 2. Relax to starting position.

8. Swim Strokes

Starter — 5 each stroke
Intermediate — 5 to 10 each stroke
Advanced — 10 to 15 each stroke

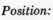

Position:
Stand erect with feet shoulder-width apart.

Count 1. Using arms only, simulate the breast stroke.
Count 2. Simulate the crawl stroke.
Count 3. Simulate the back stroke.
Count 4. Return to your starting position.

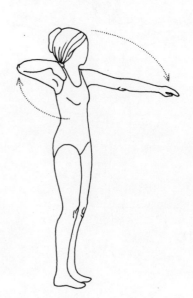

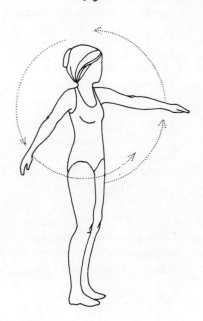

9. Half Knee Bend

Starter — Skip this exercise
Intermediate — 5 to 10 times
Advanced — 10 to 15 times

Position:
Stand erect with hands on hips.

Count 1. Bend your knees halfway while extending your arms
forward, palms down. Keep your
heels on the floor.
Count 2. Return to the starting
position.

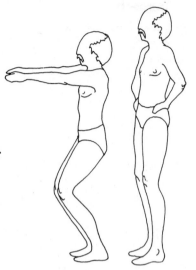

10. Shoulder Stretcher

Starter — 2 to 5 times
Intermediate — 5 to 10 times
Advanced — 10 to 20 times

Position:
Stand erect, bend arms in front
of chest with extended finger tips
touching and elbows at shoulder
height.

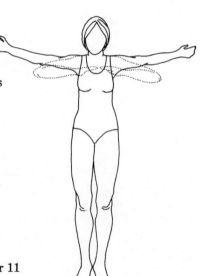

Count 1. Pull elbows back as far
as possible, then return to starting position.
Count 2. Repeat
Count 3. Repeat

At this point in the routine:
Starters walk 2 to 5 minutes.
Intermediates proceed to number 11
Advanced walk-jog for 3 minutes

11. Cat Back

All levels — 5 times

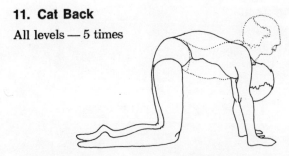

Position:
Assume a kneeling position on hands and knees.

Count 1. Arch your back upward while, at the same time, allowing your head to drop.
Count 2. Reverse this action by bringing up your head and letting your spine go swaybacked.

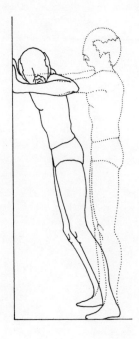

12. Standing Pushup

Intermediates only do this exercise, 10 repeats, then walk 5 minutes.

Position:
Stand erect, facing a wall, at a distance of about 18 inches, with feet about 6 inches apart, palms on the wall and bearing weight slightly.

Count 1. Allow your body to move forward toward the wall by bending your elbows. Turn your head to the side and move forward until your cheek almost touches the wall.
Count 2. Push against wall with arms returning to starting position. Try to keep heels on the floor throughout this exercise.

13. Alternate Leg Bend

Starter — 2 to 5 times
Intermediate — 5 to 10 times
Advanced — 10 to 15 times

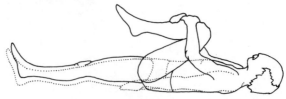

Position:
Lie on your back with legs extended and arms at your sides.

Count 1. Move left knee toward chest as far as possible; then clasp knee with both hands and pull slowly and firmly toward chest.
Count 2. Return to starting position.
Repeat this exercise with right leg.

14. Supine Stretch

Starter — 2 to 5 times
Intermediate — 5 times
Advanced — 5 times

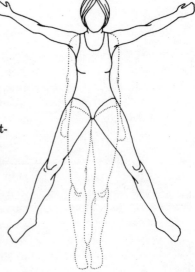

Position:
Lie on back with legs extended, feet together, arms extended at sides.

Count 1. Move arms and legs outward along the floor to a spread-eagle position. Slide your limbs; do not raise them from floor.
Count 2. Return to starting position.
Throughout this exercise, try to keep the small of the back tight against the floor by contracting the abdominal muscles.

15. Walk the Tightrope

All levels — walk 10 feet

Position:
Stand erect with left foot along a
straight line, arms extended to
aid balance.

Count 1. Walk the length of the
line by alternately placing one foot
in front of the other, toe to heel.
Count 2. Return to the starting
point by walking backward along
the line in the same manner.

At this point in the routine,
starters do half knee bends
(number 9), repeating 2 to 5
times. Then, do standing pushups (number 12), repeating 2 to
10 times. Skip exercises 16 and
17; move to 18.

16. Hop

Advanced only — 5 times on each foot.

17. Kneeling Pushup

Intermediate — 1 to 3 times
Advanced — 3 to 6 times

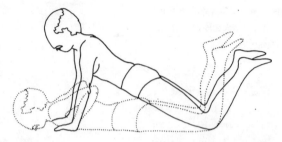

Position:
Lie prone on the floor with legs together and knees bent, feet raised off floor, hands on floor under shoulders, palms down.

Count 1. Push body off the floor until arms are fully extended and body describes a straight line from head to knees.
Count 2. Return to starting position.

18. Leg Raise

Starter — 2 to 5 times each leg
Intermediate — 5 to 10 times each leg
Advanced — 10 times each leg

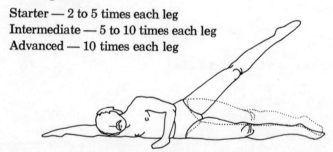

Position:
Lie with right side of your body on the floor and head resting on right arm.

Count 1. Lift your left leg sideward about 30 inches off the floor.
Count 2. Return to starting position.
Repeat with opposite side.

19. Diver's Stance

Intermediate only — hold for 10
seconds.

Position:
Stand erect with arms at sides
and feet slightly apart.

Count 1. Rise up on your toes
and bring arms upward and forward so that they extend parallel
with the floor, palms down.
Close your eyes and hold the
balance for 10 seconds.

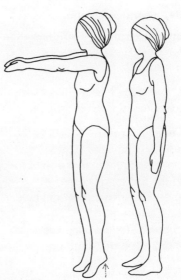

20. Abdominal Curl

Starter — 2 to 5 times, hold for 4 seconds
Intermediate — 5 times, hold for 6 seconds
Advanced — 5 times, hold for 10 seconds

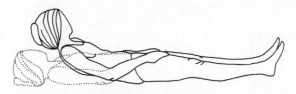

Position:
Lie on your back with legs straight, feet together and arms of
starters extended along the front of the legs with palms resting
lightly on the thighs. Intermediates cross arms over the chest.
Advanced clasp hands behind the neck.

Count 1. Tighten abdominal muscles and lift head and shoulders
so that the shoulders are about 10 inches off the floor. Hold for the
specified number of seconds.
Count 2. Return slowly to starting position, keeping abdominal
muscles tight until head and shoulders reach the floor.

21. Stork Stand

Advanced only — hold position
for 10 seconds on each leg.

Position:
Stand erect, feet slightly apart,
hands on hips, head straight.

Count 1. Transfer weight to the
left foot and bend right knee,
bringing the sole of the right foot
to the inner side of the left
knee. Close your eyes and hold
for 10 seconds.
Count 2. Repeat the exercise,
standing on the right foot.

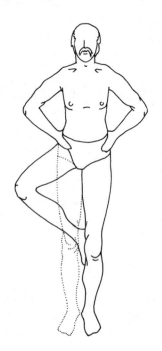

22. Walk-Jog

Starter — Walk 50 steps, jog 10 steps, 1 to 3 minutes
Intermediate — Walk 50 steps, jog 25, 3 to 6 minutes
Advanced — Walk 50 steps, jog 50 steps. Increase to walk 100
steps, jog 100 steps. Continue for 5 minutes.

23. Cool-down Walk

Starter — Walk 1 to 3 minutes.
Intermediate — Walk 1 to 3 minutes
Advanced — Walk 3 minutes.

13

Aqua Dynamics

I will go back to the great sweet mother,
Mother and lover of men, the sea.
                                    EPES SARGEANT
                              A Life on the Ocean Wave

A FITNESS CENTER IN YOUR BACK YARD

Swimming is an excellent activity for both younger and older
people. It has been estimated that there are close to 2 million
swimming pools in the United States. Of these, the vast majority are residential pools. The rest are in hotels, motels,
schools, camps, Ys, public and private clubs, and recreation
areas. In many cases, the term *swimming pool* is a misnomer
when applied to the residential variety. Few back yard pools
are larger than 36 feet long by 17 feet wide; many are considerably smaller. For an adult, a "swim" in such a pool means
diving in, gliding across to the other side, and climbing out.
Not exactly your Olympic workout. Many people consider the
back yard pool to be a great place to sit around with a drink
while watching the kids splashing about. Here we are, being
spectators again.

Actually, there's a great potential in the family swimming
pool as an exercise and conditioning opportunity. Of course, it
would be absurd to attempt a standard workout — swimming
laps, for example — in a pool resembling an oversize bathtub.
But a pool can be all you need for a complete exercise program.

I mean *complete:* cardiorespiratory endurance, muscle tone and strength development, and a marvelous routine for improving flexibility and the full range of body motion for all the muscles and joints, and you don't even have to know how to swim to do most of the exercises. The Aqua Dynamics program was developed by C. Carson Conrad, executive director of the President's Council on Physical Fitness and Sports. "Casey" Conrad, an authentic missionary for health and fitness, can be an inspiration for any older American. At the age of 64, Casey, who runs and swims several miles each day, has the body of a man thirty years younger, and the energy of a whole room full of six-year-olds. "Swimming is recognized as America's most popular active sport," says Conrad. It is an activity that can be used for recreation on one day, physical fitness on the next, and survival on another.

A GROWTH OPPORTUNITY FOR EVERYONE

The remarkable thing about swimming and Aqua Dynamics is that they are among the best physical activities for people of all ages. Aqua Dynamics is a highly recommended program for youngsters whose bodies are developing. It promotes strong supple limbs, coordination, and a sense of confidence and control in the water. The unique value of the Aqua Dynamics program is that it is a self-regulating system of activities that provide just the right amount of conditioning to meet the needs of each individual. Vigorous water activities can make a contribution to the flexibility, strength, and circulatory endurance of just about everyone. It's a great way to get even the infirm, the convalescing patient, the arthritis and rheumatism victim off the sideline and back in the game.

With the body submerged in water, blood circulation increases; pressure of the water on the body promotes relaxation and deeper ventilation of the lungs; and with the well-planned activities of the Aqua Dynamics program, circulation, relaxation, and ventilation are increased still more.

Flexibility routines are performed more easily in the water because the effects of gravity are greatly diminished. A person immersed in water up to the neck experiences an apparent loss of up to 90 percent of his or her body weight. This means, for example, that the feet and legs of a woman weighing 130 pounds would have to support the equivalent of only 13 pounds while her body is immersed in water. The effect of putting most of one's weight aside while submerged in water makes it possible for even elderly people or people with painful joints or weak leg muscles to move easily and comfortably. Most exercises are much easier to perform in the water than on the floor. Even more important, people who could never engage in such activities as jogging on dry land can enjoy the benefits of this excellent cardiorespiratory conditioner by jogging in the swimming pool.

How to Use Aqua Dynamics

A medical examination is advised before one begins any exercise or conditioning program. This aquatic routine has been designed for the basically healthy individual. One who is elderly or who suffers from a muscle or joint ailment should review the Aqua Dynamics exercises with his or her physician or physical therapist. A health professional can determine how the exercises might be used to best advantage without risk of undue exertion or strain.

Exercise programs of all kinds should be adapted to each person's tolerance level — the level at which he or she can perform comfortably and without distress. In order for Aqua Dynamics workouts to be comfortable and productive of the maximum training effect, a combination system of training should be employed using both "change of activity" and "change of pace." *Change of activity* means shifting from one activity to another, each exercise using a different set of muscles. *Change of pace* is sometimes called interval training. It means interspersing periods of more intense physical activity with recovery periods during which activity of reduced intensity is performed.

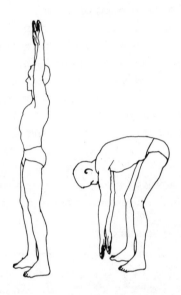

Warming Up

I have mentioned several times in previous chapters that warming up before intense exercise is a must. Warm-ups are equally important before one engages in Aqua Dynamics or any water exercises. Deck exercises can include the simulation of the various swimming strokes: the crawl, forward and reverse butterfly, breast stroke, and back stroke. These can be done at increasing degrees of intensity, accompanied by deep breathing, until a state of light perspiration occurs.

Because most swimming exercises cause the back to be in a hyperextended position, specific stretching exercises should be done at the beginning and end of each workout. A good way to stretch the back muscles and the muscles at the backs of the thighs is to follow this simple outline. Begin by standing in a relaxed position with your hands hanging by your sides and your feet slightly apart. Bring your arms forward and raise them high above your head. Reach as high as possible and hold that position for 5 to 10 seconds. Then bring your trunk forward and down while slightly flexing your knees. This puts you in a modified, bent-knee, toe-touch position. It is not necessary to actually touch your toes unless it is comfortable to do so. Hold this position for 20 to 30 seconds; then repeat the entire sequence 2 or 3 times (see Illustration 1).

Through proper warm-up, the body's deep muscle temperature is raised and the ligaments and connecting tissues stretched. This prepares the body for vigorous activity and helps to prevent injury and discomfort.

The following Aqua Dynamics program can be done in a small residential pool or in a corner or limited area of a crowded institutional pool.

STANDING WATER DRILLS

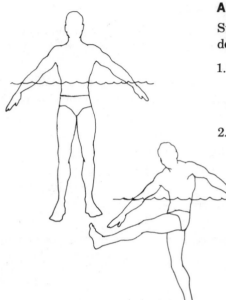

Alternate Toe Touch

Standing in waist-to-chest-deep water,

1. Raise left leg, bringing right hand toward left foot, with left arm extended rearward.
2. Recover to starting position.
   Repeat in reverse.

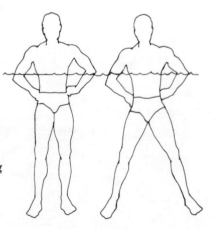

Side Straddle Hop

Standing in waist-to-chest-deep water with hands on hips,

1. Jump sideward, positioning feet approximately two feet apart.
2. Recover.

Stride Hop

Standing in waist-to-chest-
deep water with hands on
hips,

1. Jump, with left leg forward
   and right leg back.
2. Jump, changing to right leg
   forward and left leg back.
   Repeat.

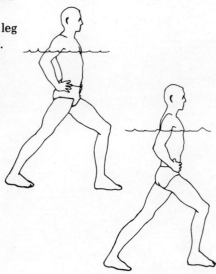

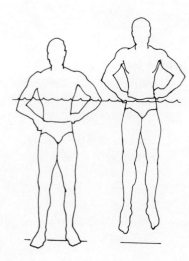

Toe Bounce

Standing in waist-to-chest-
deep water with hands on hips,
jump with feet together
through a bouncing move-
ment of the feet.
Repeat.

Rise on Toes

Standing in chest-deep water,

1. Raise up on toes.
2. Lower to starting position.
   Repeat and accelerate.

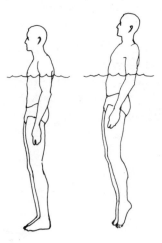

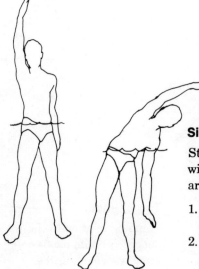

Side Bender

Standing in waist-deep water, with left arm at side and right arm over head,

1. Stretch, slowly bending to the left.
2. Recover to starting position.
   Repeat, reversing to right arm at side and left arm over head.

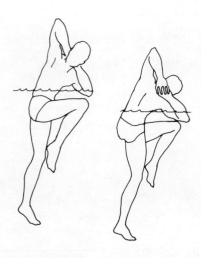

Walking Twists

Standing in waist-to-chest-deep water and with fingers laced behind neck, walk forward, bringing up alternate legs, twisting body to touch knee with opposite elbow. Repeat.

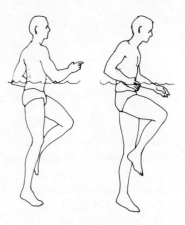

Jogging in Place

Standing in chest-deep water with arms bent in running position, jog in place.

Standing Crawl

Standing in waist-to-chest-deep water, simulate the overhand crawl stroke by:

1. Reaching out with the left hand, getting a grip on the water, pressing downward and pulling, bringing the left hand through to the thigh.
2. Reaching out with the right hand, etc. Repeat.

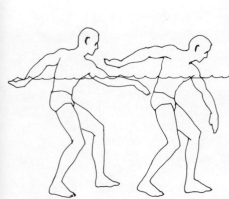

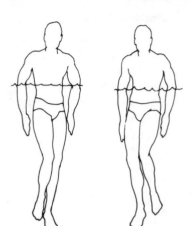

Bouncing

Standing in chest-deep water,

1. Bounce on left foot, at the same time pushing down vigorously with both hands, causing the body to rise.
2. Bounce on left foot, etc.

Bounding in Place with Alternate Arm Stretched Forward

Standing in waist-deep water,

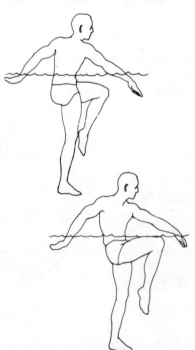

1. Bound in place with high knee action; right arm is outstretched far forward when left knee is high. Left arm and hand are stretched rearward.
2. Bring the right knee high, with the left arm and hand outstretched forward. The right arm and hand are stretched rearward.

Special note: When the position of the arms is reversed, pull down and through the water with hand, simulating the propulsion of the crawl stroke.

Repeat.

POOL-SIDE STANDING DRILLS

Stretch and Touch

Standing at side of pool in
waist-to-chest-deep water,
facing wall with arms ex-
tended and fingertips approximately 12 inches from wall,

1. With shoulder under water
   twist left and try to touch
   wall with both hands.
2. Twist right and try to touch
   wall with both hands.
   Repeat.

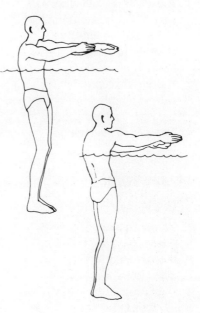

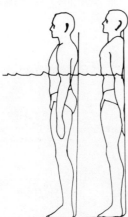

Flat Back

Standing at side of pool in
waist-to-chest-deep water,

1. Press back against wall,
   holding for 6 counts.
2. Relax to starting position.
   Repeat.

Pull and Stretch

Standing at side of pool with
back against the wall,

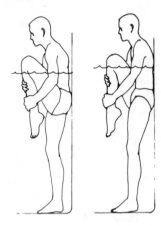

1. Raise left leg and clasp calf
   with both arms, pulling leg
   vigorously to chest.
2. Recover to starting position.
3. Raise right leg and clasp
   calf with both arms, pulling
   leg vigorously to chest.
4. Recover to starting position.

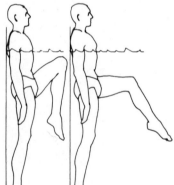

Leg Out

Standing at side of pool in
chest-deep water with back
against the wall,

1. Raise left knee to chest.
2. Extend left leg straight out.
3. Stretch leg.
4. Drop leg to starting position.

   Repeat, reversing to right
   leg.

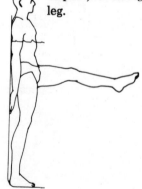

GUTTER-HOLDING DRILLS

Pool Side, Knees Up

Supine, holding on to pool
gutter with hands and with
legs extended,

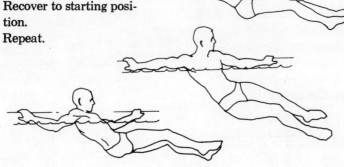

1. Bring knees to chin.
2. Recover to starting position.
   Repeat.

Twisting Legs

Supine, holding on to pool
gutter, with legs extended,

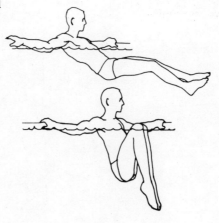

1. Twist slowly to left.
2. Recover.
3. Twist slowly to right.
4. Recover.
   Repeat.

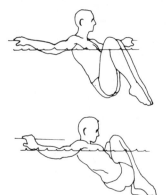

Knees Up, Twisting

Supine, holding on to pool gutter, with knees drawn up to chest,

1. Twist slowly to left.
2. Recover.
3. Twist slowly to right.
4. Recover.
   Repeat.

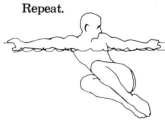

Leg Crosses

Supine, holding on to pool gutter, with legs extended,

1. Swing legs far apart.
2. Bring legs together, crossing left leg over right.
3. Swing legs far apart.
4. Bring legs together, crossing right leg over left.
   Repeat.

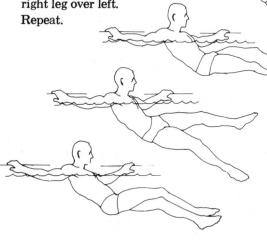

Twist Hips

Standing, holding on to pool
gutter, with back to wall,

1. Twist hips to left as far as
   possible, keeping the upper
   trunk facing forward.
2. Recover.
3. Twist hips to right.
4. Recover.

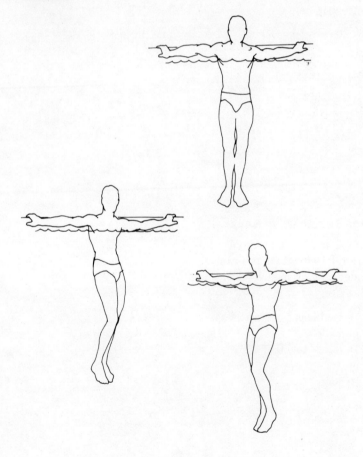

Alternate Raised-Knee Crossovers

Standing, holding on to pool gutter, with back to wall,

1. Lift left knee and cross it over; twist to right.
2. Recover.
3. Lift right knee and cross it over; twist to left.
4. Recover.
   Repeat.

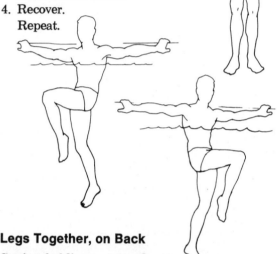

Legs Together, on Back

Supine, holding on to pool gutter, legs together and extended about 6 inches under the water,

1. Spread legs as far apart as possible.
2. Pull legs together vigorously.
   Repeat.

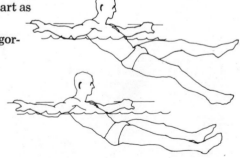

Legs Together, on Front

Prone, holding on to pool gutter with one hand flat on
wall, push legs out, with feet
together,

1. Spread legs as far apart as
   possible.
2. Pull legs together vigorously.
   Repeat.

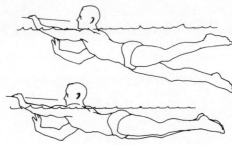

Raising Hips

Prone, holding on to pool
gutter with one hand flat on
wall, push legs out,

1. Raise hips, holding for 4
   counts.
2. Relax.
   Repeat.

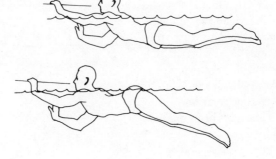

Circle Legs

Prone, holding on to pool gutter with one hand flat on
wall, push legs out,

1. Circle legs outward right.
2. Repeat.
3. Reverse to right.
4. Repeat.

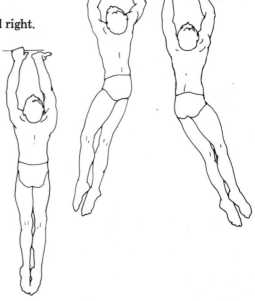

Elementary Bobbing

Standing in shallow water,

1. Take a breath.
2. Submerge in a tuck position
   with feet on the pool bottom. Exhale during steps
   2 and 3.
3. Shove up off the bottom of
   the pool and regain a
   standing position.
4. Inhale with head out of
   water.
5. Repeat 1, 2, 3, and 4.

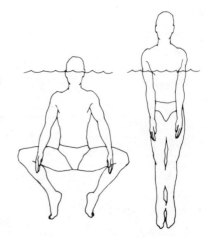

Leg Swing Outward

Standing with back against
side of pool and hands holding gutter,

1. Raise left leg as high as
   possible with leg straight.
2. Swing foot and leg to left
   side.
3. Recover to starting position
   by pulling left leg vigorously to right.
   Repeat.
4. Reverse to right leg.
   Repeat.

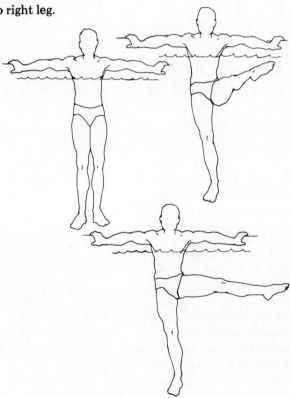

Alternate Leg, Rearward Bobbing

Standing in shallow water,

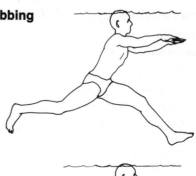

1. Take a breath.
2. Submerge with left leg in a squatting position, left foot on pool bottom and right leg extended rearward. Exhale during 2 and 3.
3. Shove up off the bottom and reverse the position of the legs, breathing while the head is out of water.
4. Submerge with right leg in a squatting position, right foot on pool bottom and left leg extended rearward. Exhale during the action.
   Repeat 1, 2, 3, and 4.

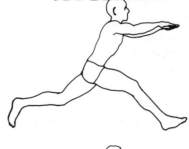

Legs Astride Bobbing

Standing in waist-to-chest-deep water,

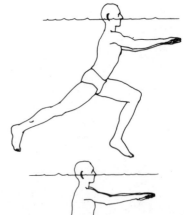

1. Take a breath.
2. Submerge with legs astride, left leg forward, right leg rearward. Exhale during 2 and 3.
3. Shove off bottom, inhale when head is out of water.
4. Submerge with legs astride, reversing legs. Exhale during action.
   Repeat.

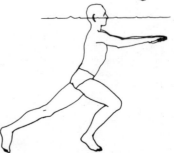

Alternate Leg, Sideward Bobbing

Standing in waist-to-chest-
deep water,

1. Take a breath.
2. Submerge with left leg in
   a full squatting position,
   left foot on pool bottom and
   right leg extended sideward. Exhale during 2 and 3.
3. Shove off bottom, reversing
   the position of the legs and
   inhaling while head is out
   of water.
4. Submerge with the right
   leg in a full squatting position, right foot on pool
   bottom and the left leg
   extended sideward. Exhale
   during the action.
   Repeat.

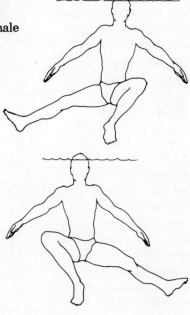

Progressive Alternate Leg, Forward Bobbing

Standing, swimmer: performs action described in Alternate Leg, Rearward Bobbing, alternating legs bobbing progressively, and moving forward the length of the pool or a specified distance.

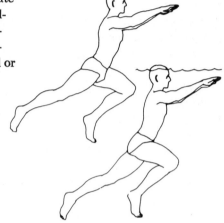

Advanced Bobbing

Treading in deep water, swimmer:

1. Assumes a vertical position with arms extended outward from the sides, just under the surface of the water, with palms turned down. Legs are drawn up in a position of readiness for a frog or scissors kick as arms are extended over head allowing body to sink.
2. Executes kick as hands are pulled sharply to thighs. (As a result of this action, the head and shoulders rise out of the water and a deep breath is taken at the highest point.)
3. As the body sinks, exhales and stretches the arms over head.
   Repeat.

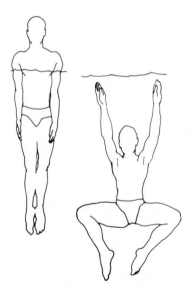

Progressive "Bunny Hop" Bobbing

Standing, swimmer:

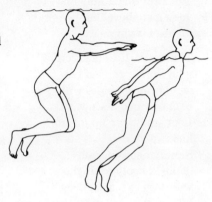

1. Takes a breath.
2. Submerges in a tuck or full squatting position with feet on pool bottom.
3. Pushes up and forward off bottom of pool, exhaling during 2 and 3.
4. Inhales with head out of water.
5. Repeat, pushing forward the length of the pool or specified distance.

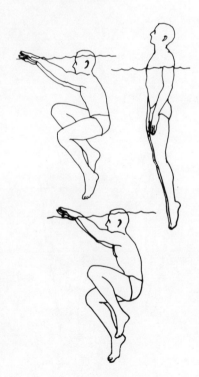

Left/Right Leg Bobbing

Standing or treading in deep water, swimmer:

1. Takes a breath.
2. Submerges in a tuck, with right leg drawn up and left foot on pool bottom.
3. Pushes upward with left leg thrust. Exhales during 2 and 3.
4. Inhales with head out of water.
5. Repeat, reversing action of legs.

High Bobbing

In water approximately one to three feet above the swimmer's head, swimmer:

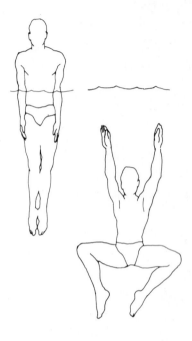

1. Takes a vertical position with arms extended outward from the sides with palms turned downward. Legs are drawn up for frog kick.
2. Simultaneously, pulls hands sharply to thighs with legs executing frog kick.
3. Inhales at peak of height.
4. Drops with thrust of arms upward, palms turned upward, until feet reach bottom of pool and tucks to a squat position. Exhales throughout this action.
5. Jumps upward with power leg thrust, at the same time pulling arms downward in a breast stroke motion, causing the head and shoulders to rise high out of the water. Exhales during 4 and 5.
6. Inhales and repeats cycles 4 and 5, etc.

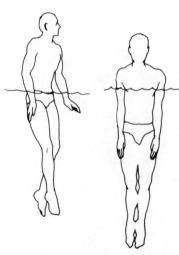

Power Bobbing

Power bobbing is similar to "high bobbing" except that at the top of the upward thrust the hands scull (see instructions for sculling on page 139) vigorously as the legs flutter kick. In "power bobbing" the swimmer will literally blast out of the water, exposing all of the body down to the hips. Power bobbing is a well-rounded workout involving leg power, arm and shoulder work, heavy forced breathing, and rhythmical action.

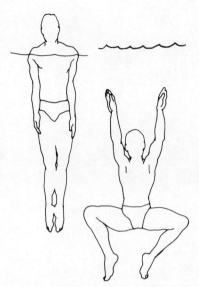

TREADING WATER

Elementary Treading

In water deep enough that toes will not touch bottom in a perpendicular position, swimmer sculls or fins as he kicks . . . bicycle, scissors, or frog style.

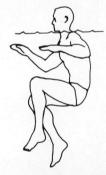

Advanced Treading

In water over his head in a perpendicular position, swimmer kicks bicycle, scissors, or frog style with hands held shoulder high.

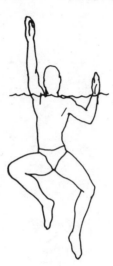

One-Hand-High Treading

In water over his head in a perpendicular position, swimmer:

1. Kicks bicycle, scissors, or frog style, holding one arm straight up and other hand shoulder high.
2. Reverses arms.

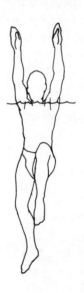

Two-Hands-High Treading

In water over his head in a perpendicular position, swimmer kicks bicycle, scissors, or frog style holding both arms straight up out of water.

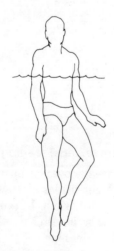

Lookout Treading

In water over his head in a perpendicular position, swimmer kicks vigorously, at the same time thrashing the water by sculling. This raises the shoulders and chest high out of the water.

EXTENSIONS

Breathing. Controlled breathing is essential for the activities that follow. The swimmer should inhale through the mouth and exhale through the nose. One should be exhaling through the nose any time the head is underwater.

Skulling. "Extension" activities are largely dependent on one's skulling ability. Skulling is done by arm and hand action; it can provide lifting force or combined lifting and propulsion force. The use of the hands and arms in skulling is the same basic action regardless of the position of the body or the direction one wishes the body to move. The swimmer soon learns the slight variations of force and hand position that result in lateral movement. Basically, though, the swimmer is attempting to suspend himself in deep water with his head remaining above the surface (unless otherwise specified). The skulling action usually begins by pushing the palms downward and away from one another, with the thumbs pointed slightly downward, until the arms are almost extended at the sides. Then, the palms are pulled forward and toward one another with the wrists rotated so that the thumbs point slightly upward. The movements are done alternately. Within a very short period of time, the swimmer will automatically adjust the angle of the palms and the force of the arm movements so that the necessary amount of upward thrust is produced.

Special note: On all "extension" activities that follow, the swimmer should endeavor to stay in one place in the pool.

Left Knee Up and Back

Assuming a supine position, swimmer:

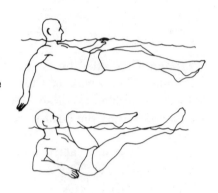

1. Sculls, drawing left knee up to chest with right knee extended and toes on the right foot out of water.
2. Sculls, straightening the left leg, thus returning to the starting position. Repeats.

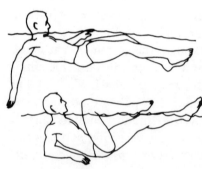

Right Knee Up and Back

Assuming a supine position, swimmer:

1. Sculls, drawing right leg up to chest with left leg extended and toes on the left foot out of water.
2. Sculls, straightening the right leg, thus returning to the starting position. Repeats.

Knees Up and Back

Starting from a supine position, swimmer:

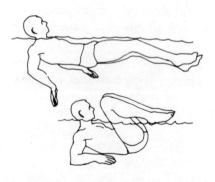

1. Sculls, drawing knees up to chest.
2. Sculls, shoving legs forward and returning to a back-lying position. Repeats.

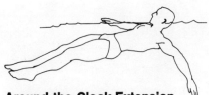

Around-the-Clock Extension

Starting from a horizontal position, swimmer:

1. Sculls, drawing knees up
   to chest, shoving legs forward to a back-lying position.
2. Sculls vigorously, drawing
   legs up to chest, shoving
   legs to left side, causing
   the body to be in a right
   side-stroke position.
3. Sculls vigorously, drawing
   knees up to chest and then
   shoving legs out to a front-
   lying position.
4. Sculls vigorously, drawing
   knees up to chest, shoving
   legs to right side, causing
   the body to be in a left
   side-stroke position.
   Repeats.

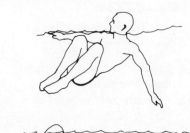

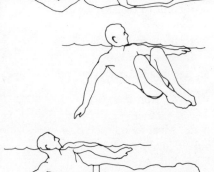

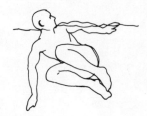

OTHER WATER EXERCISES

Pedaling in Water

Starting from a back-lying position, swimmer simulates a
pedaling motion with knees
raised alternately to the chest.
Uses reverse sculling to remain in same place in the
pool.

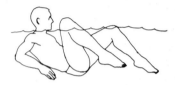

Left-Leg Raiser

Starting from a back-lying position, swimmer:

1. Sculls continuously, bringing left knee to chest until
   knee is almost parallel to
   surface of the water.
2. Sculls, straightening the
   left leg until it is perpendicular to the surface of
   water.
3. Returns to 1, the left-knee-
   to-chest position.
4. Returns to back-lying position.
   Repeats.

Note: Most men find it difficult to achieve a full vertical
leg extension.

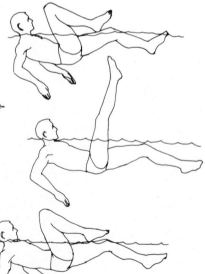

Rub-a-Dub-Dub

Starting from a back-lying position, swimmer brings knees to chest, with knees and toes together.

1. Spins in a circle, using an opposite sculling motion of hands.
2. After one full turn, reverses action.
   Repeats.

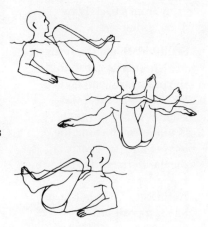

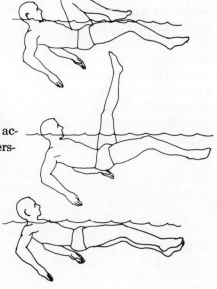

Right-Leg Raiser

Starting from a back-lying position, swimmer repeats actions of *left-leg raiser*, reversing position of legs.

Alternate Leg Raiser

Starting from a back-lying position, swimmer:

1. Sculls continuously, bringing left knee to chest until thigh is nearly perpendicular to the surface of the water.
2. Sculls, straightening the left leg until it is perpendicular to the surface of the water.
3. Returns to 1, the left-knee-to-chest position.
4. Returns to back-lying position.
5. Sculls continuously, bringing right knee to chest as in 1.
6. Sculls, straightening the right leg until it is perpendicular to the surface of the water.
7. Returns to 5, the right-knee-to-chest position.
8. Returns to back-lying position. Continue alternating left and right action.

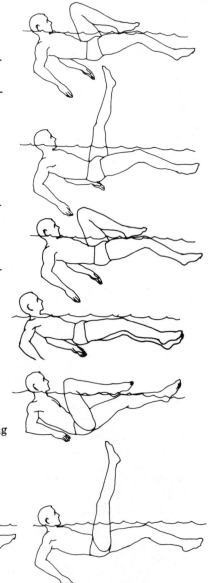

Double Leg Raiser

Starting from a back-lying position, swimmer:

1. Sculls continuously, bringing knees to chest until thighs are almost perpendicular to the water.
2. Straightens both legs together, extending them skyward so that they are nearly perpendicular to the surface of the water.
3. Returns to the back-lying position.
   Repeats.

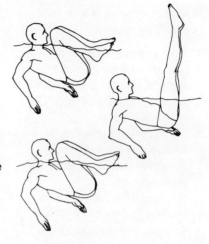

High Sculling

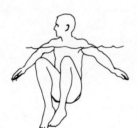

Starting from a standing position, swimmer brings knees to chest with heels close to hips and sculls, figure-8 motion, vigorously using arms only, raising the upper body as high as possible out of the water.

Under and Up

Swim 4 breast strokes under water, come up and breathe. Repeat.

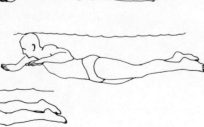

Alternate Treading and Sculling

In deep water and in a vertical
position, swimmer:

1. Treads water with hands
   held shoulder high and the
   body in a vertical position
   for as long as is comfortably
   possible.
2. Shifts to sculling action of
   the arms and hands, with
   the knees pulled up so that
   heels are under the hips.
   Sculling without the use of
   the legs is done for as long
   as is comfortably possible.

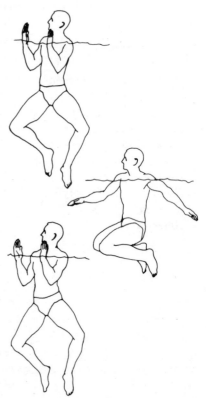

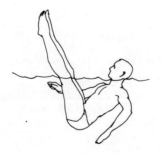

Sculling V Sit

From a back-lying position,
lower hips and raise feet out of
the water with toes pointed so
that the body is in a V position,
and scull in the direction the
swimmer is facing. Maintain for
as long as is comfortably possible.

LAP SWIMMING

Despite the small distance covered after the shove-off and glide in the residential pool, lap swimming can still be an excellent activity. If the pool is clear, take off and enjoy swimming hard until you begin to feel winded. Ease off by loafing with a lazy breast stroke or side stroke until you feel recovered, then go again. Another way to begin an interval training program in the swimming pool is to swim one length of the pool, get out, walk back, and repeat a number of times. For an individual in poor physical condition following a regimen of 5 to 10 lengths, walking back after each length, may be necessary for several weeks or months. As endurance increases, the number of lengths should be increased progressively.

WORKOUTS

In order to illustrate how the exercises described in the Aqua Dynamics program can be combined in different workouts, the following examples are provided:

VERY LOW GEAR ... 15 MINUTES

Side Straddle Hop	15 seconds
Standing Crawl	30 seconds
Walking Twists	15 seconds
Toe Bounce	15 seconds
Flat Back	15 seconds
Pull and Stretch	30 seconds
Leg Out	30 seconds
Front Flutter	30 seconds
Back Flutter	30 seconds
Alternate Leg, Rearward Bobbing	1 minute
Leg Swing Outward	30 seconds

Bounding in Place with Arm Stretch	30 seconds
Elementary Treading	30 seconds
Lap Swimming	9 minutes

Low Gear ... 20 Minutes

Stride Hop	15 seconds
Standing Crawl	30 seconds
Front Flutter	1 minute
Back Flutter	1 minute
Front Flutter	1 minute
Pull and Stretch	30 seconds
Leg Swing Outward	1 minute
Advanced Bobbing	1 minute
Left Knee Up and Back	30 seconds
Right Knee Up and Back	30 seconds
Alternate Leg, Rearward Bobbing	30 seconds
Knees Up and Back	30 seconds
Alternate Leg, Sideward Bobbing	30 seconds
Bounding in Place with Arm Stretch	45 seconds
Knees Up and Front	30 seconds
Advanced Bobbing	1 minute
Knee Up, Left	30 seconds
Knees Up, Right	30 seconds
Advanced Bobbing	1 minute
Reverse Sides Extension	30 seconds
Lap Swimming — Interval	6½ minutes

Middle Gear ... 30 Minutes

Front Flutter	2 minutes
Back Flutter	2 minutes
Front Flutter	1 minute
Alternate Leg, Rearward Bobbing	1 minute
Knees Up and Front	1 minute
Knees Up and Back	1 minute
Alternate Leg, Sideward Bobbing	1 minute
Front and Back Extensions	1 minute
High Bobbing	3 minutes
Reverse Sides Extension	1 minute

Progressive Bobbing	2 minutes
Rub-a-Dub-Dub	2 minutes
Left-Leg Raiser	15 seconds
Right-Leg Raiser	15 seconds
Alternate Leg Raisers	30 seconds
High Bobbing	1 minute
Lap Swimming — Interval	10 minutes

HIGH GEAR ... 60 MINUTES

Front Flutter	3 minutes
Back Flutter	3 minutes
Advanced Bobbing	3 minutes
Left Knee Up and Back	1 minute
Right Knee Up and Back	1 minute
Knees Up and Back	1 minute
High Bobbing	3 minutes
Knees Up and Front	1 minute
Alternate Leg, Rearward Bobbing	2 minutes
Front and Back Extensions	2 minutes
Alternate Leg, Sideward Bobbing	2 minutes
Reverse Sides Extensions	2 minutes
Bounding in Place with Arm Stretch	3 minutes
Progressive Alternate Leg, Forward Bobbing	3 minutes
Rub-a-Dub-Dub	3 minutes
Left Leg Raiser	30 seconds
Right Leg Raiser	30 seconds
Power Bobbing	1 minute
Alternate Leg Raisers	30 seconds
Bounding in Place with Arm Stretch	3 minutes
Toe Bounce	1½ minutes
Leg Swing Outward	2 minutes
Lap Swimming	18 minutes

BUILD UP SLOWLY

The key to success in any exercise program is to build up slowly to higher levels of activity. Remember that staying in the game is predicated on growth, being a little bit better today than yesterday. Many people who have allowed themselves to lapse into a state of poor physical condition will be inspired by this book and by other sources to attempt to reunite the divided dimensions of their lives . . . to bring the physical, the mental, and the spiritual components into harmony. But consider that it probably took years, perhaps the better part of a lifetime, to become out of shape and completely split off from the body. The Aqua Dynamics program can be a pleasant and rewarding way to rediscover the athlete within you, but proceed slowly. Be satisfied with that small portion of daily growth that truly is growth.

14

The Role of Play

Here, then, we have the first main characteristic of
play: that it is free; is, in fact, freedom.

JOHAN HUIZINGA
*Homo Ludens: A Study of the
Play-Element in Culture*

Implicit in our stated goal, to stay in the game, is the acceptance of the game as life's metaphor. George Leonard calls
it the *game of games*. "The playground," says Leonard in *The
Ultimate Athlete*, "the magic circle, for this particular game
is the planet earth. The overall game time is the period between conception and death." Lest the reader see Leonard's
proposition as facetious or, at the least, tenuous, one should
point out that he qualifies it: "To say 'life is a game' is to
imply something beyond life which is not a game. This 'something,' imagined or real, undoubtedly does exist."

For some of us, perceiving life as a game is a tough psychological reach. But the idea of "staying in the game" as a
philosophical base for mental and physical fitness is quite
acceptable and attractive. Play, then, is presented as a dimension of our training program, as an avenue to both physical
and mental fitness. Into play we can invest total concentration, maximum effort, and supreme dedication, and then, not
have to be responsible for our actions. What a release! Play
can also provide a time of dissociation, little effort, and perhaps next to no concentration at all. It is either a game with

defined rules and boundaries or it is doing almost anything in a playful manner.

Our interest is in play that has a physical component, that brings us fitness as a by-product rather than as an end in itself. As we begin to arrange the components of our training program, we are going to learn some things about ourselves. One of the crucial things we must know about ourselves is this: What kind of training are we capable of doing on a permanent basis? Some of us need structure in our lives and the more directions there are in our program, the more comfortable we feel. Others need clearly defined goals and objectives and, along with these, we may look for or assign specific rewards. Then, there are those who are "turned off" by structures or systems. All of these concepts apply to fitness programs. Jack may find that the walk-jog-run program in this book is just right for him. It gives a system for upgrading his cardiorespiratory fitness that is easy to follow, yet is specific without having too many charts or numbers. Anne, an electronics engineer, likes Dr. Cooper's aerobics program because of its mathematic neatness: So many minutes, so many miles, so many times a week equals a specific level of fitness for a person of a certain age.

Then there are those who, like George Sheehan, have to find their fitness in their play. For such individuals, a run or a swim or a bike ride each day has nothing to do with miles or minutes. It is play; therefore it becomes addictive, it becomes necessary. Because it is necessary, a new lifestyle evolves around it. Dr. Sheehan compares pure exercise and play exercise like this: "Exercise is something that has no meaning — that is done for a purpose. Play is something we do because it has meaning ... but it has no purpose." Let's take a closer look at that.

I often run in Brookdale Park in Montclair, New Jersey. The park includes several acres of rolling meadows and wooded areas with footpaths and roadways. In the center of the park is a quarter-mile cinder track. Running the track every morn-

tally and physically in much the way college football had.
He did not decide on table tennis. Wally found a rugby league,
and that became his passion. Although he runs to keep himself in shape, he does not consider himself a runner. He doesn't
have the body of a marathoner. On the other hand, I spent
some time with Frank Shorter at Dr. Ken Cooper's Aerobics
Center in Dallas. Frank, one of the world's finest distance
runners and a former Olympic Gold Medal winner, is only a
couple of inches shorter than Wally Maher, but he weighs
about 90 pounds less. He has the ideal marathoner's body —
long, lean, light-boned, and no fat. But Frank would never be-
long on a football or rugby field.

Today, a growing number of physical educators are attempting to use body typing as a better way to classify students
and, ultimately, to guide them into exercise and play activities
that are compatible with their physiologies. The pioneering
work on body typing (somatotyping) was done by William H.
Sheldon, Ph.D., M.D., a scientist distinguished by an almost
poet-like insight into his science. In his classic work, *Atlas of
Men*, Dr. Sheldon revealed that insight:

> We are still being born into a world of such beauty as stag-
> gers the imagination and beggars speech, and the physical real-
> ity that man is carries the stamp of truth even when the beauty
> is obscure to perception. In such a world it seems reasonable to
> suppose that there should be a way of so truthfully reflecting a
> man's structural self that the reflection will blend with the con-
> tinuum of order like faint music. The somatotype is therefore a
> groping for a reflection in man of the orderly continuum of
> nature and, in a more specific way, it is also an attempt to iden-
> tify the music of one's own particular dance of life.

Dr. Sheldon was convinced that the body told all and that
within certain limits the three classic body configurations
really constituted the three great races of man. Each body
type has its characteristic personality, Sheldon believed, and
its characteristic way of dealing with the world. Sheldon broke
down the three body types as follows:

ing are Dr. Cooper's exercise types with their stopwatche
pacing off the miles. Each of them has a purpose — fitnes
The miles around the track are simply the method. They ha
no meaning. Ambling along the shaded footpaths we fi
many of Dr. Sheehan's "play-types." Some of them may ha
gotten into running with fitness as the objective but somethi
happened. The run itself became paramount. The medi
became the message. For such runners, the meaning, the j
the play is in the run; the purpose has receded.

Of course, this thinking applies to any fitness or play
tivity. The trouble with it is that it requires a certain de
of self-knowledge. We are all familiar with the reasons pe
offer for dropping out of fitness programs. Often it is bec
they are square pegs forcing themselves into round holes.
person who needs a structured, by-the-numbers type of
gram will not usually find the discipline to achieve fi
purely through play activities. Likewise, an individual
could easily get caught up in running or walking or cy
may balk at the regimentation of an organized prograr
troverts enjoy doing things with other people, whether
pure exercise or a sports activity. Introverted people u
tend toward solitary exercise or play activity. The "lon
of the long distance runner" is a very well known con
these days, although most distance runners would pr
substitute the word *solitude* for loneliness.

Other factors influence the kinds of play activities
dividual will find enjoyable. Foremost among these i
type. Each of us has a body that is made to do some
well and others not so well. Wally Maher is a radio
caster in Atlanta, using the pseudonym "Beau Bock."
who stands about six feet two and weighs in at ab
pounds, was a ferocious lineman for the University o:
football team. To look at Wally Maher is to know that
athlete; he radiates power. When Wally had been out
for a couple of years and began putting on weight, h
looking around for something that would challenge h

Endomorphs. The endomorph likes to eat. He or she has to work harder than the other body types to keep from putting on excessive weight. This type tends to become roly-poly. Dr. Sheldon assigned the endomorph the best disposition; the endomorph is outgoing and social.

Mesomorph. The mesomorph is characterized by a predominance of mesodermally derived tissue — bone, muscle, and connective tissue. He is likely to have massive strength and pronounced muscle development. The mesomorphic build represents the classic criterion for the athlete or the warrior. He is apt to be bold, hearty, and aggressive.

Ectomorph. The ectomorph is thin and wiry with a predominance of what Sheldon referred to as "ectodermally derived tissue," which is mainly the skin and "its appendages including the nervous system." Supposedly, with his greater sensory exposure to the outside world, the ectomorph is a sensitive, withdrawn individual.

In actuality, we seldom find pure specimens to illustrate these body types. Most people are "cross breeds," if you will, showing characteristics of more than one body type. But there will be dominant characteristics that may influence our choice of exercise and/or play. For example, the heavyweight boxer might be an example of the pure or nearly pure mesomorph, as would the fullback, or maybe the tight end in football. The halfback or pass receiver in football, the outfielder in baseball, and the male or female tennis star might well illustrate a mesomorph/ectomorph type. Finally, the defensive lineman in football, the catcher on a baseball team, and the sumo wrestler would be samples of the mesomorph/endomorph.

We mustn't consider this information to be restrictive; it isn't meant to dissuade any reader from attempting any particular exercise or play activity. It may help some readers make a more intelligent appraisal of exercise, play, and sports. A person with ectomorphic characteristics may find that he or she is a natural runner or walker. Someone else with more endomorphic tendencies may be more at home on a bicycle or in a swimming pool.

George Sheehan offers a simple approach to finding our play: "Think back to the things you liked to do as a child." The child quickly learns what games and physical activities result in the "freedom" that Huizinga spoke of.

Play, then, can be your fitness program or can be an adjunct to it. Tennis, racquetball, squash, hiking, skiing, and skindiving are all play activities that have a physical fitness component. But in addition to that they offer the many psychological, emotional, and spiritual benefits of play. An extraordinary remedy for stress, play contains the germ of the creative process. "Play," wrote Huizinga, "not being ordinary life, stands outside the immediate satisfaction of wants and desires." Perhaps even more important to the player, in our stress-ridden society, "Into an imperfect world and into the confusion of life it brings a temporary, a limited perfection."

Two words of caution are appropriate here. First, do not attempt to benefit or remain fit on a game or two of tennis once or twice a week. Any rigorous physical undertaking done sporadically or occasionally is not only useless as a fitness activity, it can be lethal. Our training program requires us to do something for cardiorespiratory fitness every day or at least three or four times a week. As we learned earlier, exercise must occur at a certain frequency and intensity and last for a certain length of time in order for a "training effect" to take place. A weekly game of squash or tennis or racquetball does not satisfy this requirement. If you decide that play is important to your physical, mental, and spiritual fitness, make sure that you supplement it with a *regular* exercise program unless you can indulge in your sport every day or every other day. Even then, it is important that you do not elevate your pulse rate beyond your target zone.

The second admonition I feel it necessary to mention here is: Don't play for the wrong reasons. Play is a form of recreation. It is recreation in the truest sense if we understand that the word *recreation* embraces creativity: It is "re-creation." We must be able to separate our play from the dimensions of our lives in which we feel compelled to succeed ... to win ... to show tangible results for our efforts.

A friend of mine is a very intense, successful businessman. He plays golf every Saturday. I have seen my friend turn livid with anger over a missed putt. I have seen him throw golf clubs. I have seen him stalk off the golf course and make straight for the clubhouse bar — his clubs abandoned on a fairway or putting green. When my friend plays golf, he isn't *playing*. He is engaged in a competitive must-win situation. Like so many people — especially successful business types — my friend takes all of his anxieties, competitiveness, and compulsive behavior out on the golf course with him. What he is doing does not qualify as play; it is stressful.

In seeking our play, then, we examine ourselves. We begin with the body and what it is capable of doing or capable of being trained to do. Then, we decide whether our play should be something we do alone or with others. And, finally, we return to childhood for direction. We seek out the activity that brought joy to us as children, for in that activity we will find our childhood again. The thing we loved to do as youngsters has all of the elements already built into it. It is right for us physically, mentally, and spiritually. It contains that magic dimension in which the rest of the world falls away, and for a time, it is, in fact, freedom.

IF YOU WANT TO COMPETE

Dr. George Sheehan talks about the joy of running for fitness, for a play experience, for meditation on the run. "But," he says, "for many of us that's not enough. You have to take yourself somewhere on a Sunday, enter a race, and find out who you are."

In the final analysis, that's what competition is all about:

finding out who we are. A foot race, for example, pits us against other runners, and we end up with our names listed in the order of the finish. Our time for the distance and our order of finish provide a quantitative statement as to our performance in relationship to the other runners. But the most meaningful information to emerge from the experience is the personal, internal message that tells us we have met a challenge adequately or we haven't. In a marathon perhaps 5 percent of the competitors are in contention for the winner's circle. For the rest, the act of winning over other competitors is a secondary drama — a subplot, if you will — to the personal challenge. Distance running has produced a new perception of competition in which one's fellow competitors are a backdrop to an individual's confrontation with self. And I think this can be true in any sport.

A very real need for competition seems to exist among some older Americans. Such competition provides an arena for exercising and demonstrating the qualities prized by our culture: vision, discipline, and the setting and achieving of goals. Competition causes the metaphor to come alive: The competitor is in the game.

Several avenues are open to readers who believe that they would like to engage in some form of competition. Running provides the most accessible opportunities. If you have brought your walk-jog-run program to the point at which you feel ready to do some racing, there should be a number of local races that would be within your capabilities. It would be a good idea to check in with your physician first. Then inquire at your local Y about local road races which would not be too taxing for you. If there is a Road Runners club or a jogging club in your area, they will have a complete schedule of racing dates. You may find similar opportunities for competition in cycling, swimming, and cross-country skiing. Competition will usually be based on distance or age group. This will help you stay within your limitations.

For more formalized competition, consider the opportunities offered by the Amateur Athletic Union and the Senior Olympics Program. The A.A.U. has set up a national program of age-group competition in swimming, track, and field, and in other sports. You can find out about this program by having a nearby college or high school athletic director help you to get in touch with the nearest A.A.U. regional office. The A.A.U. representative will tell you how you can get involved and provide you with a schedule of dates and locations. You can also write to:

A.A.U. International Headquarters
2400 West 86th Street
Indianapolis, Indiana 46268

The folks at A.A.U. Headquarters will be happy to refer you to your state or local association.

The Senior Olympics Program administered by Senior Sports International, Inc., a nonprofit organization in Los Angeles, provides additional, nationwide opportunities for age-group competition. Adult athletes from the age of 25 up to the 70s and 80s compete in local and national matches in sports such as:

Archery	Handball
Badminton	Harmonica
Basketball	Hockey
Body Building	Lawn Bowls
Boogie Boarding	Marathon
Bowling	Martial Arts
Canoeing/Kayaking	Ocean Aquatics
Cycling	Olympic Lifting
Decathlon	Paddle Tennis
Diving	Photography
Fencing	Power Lifting
Frisbee	Racquetball
Gymnastics	Recreational Ice Skating

Rifle	Tennis
Roller Skating	Track/Field
Rugby	Volleyball
Sailing	Water Polo
Shuffleboard	Wrestling
Skill Boxing	Winter Sports:
Skin Diving	Alpine Skiing
Soccer	X-C Skiing
Softball	Speed Skating
Swimming	

The Senior Olympics program is the result of a commitment to fitness for the entire population on the part of fitness pioneer Warren Blaney, who has graciously invited readers of this book to correspond with him if they are interested in competition. He will tell you how to become a member of the Senior Olympics, how to participate in local, regional, and national events and how to set up a Senior Olympics Program in your community. "It's fantastic," Warren says. "We have people in their 70s and 80s running, jumping, pole vaulting." You can write to Warren Blaney at the following address:

Warren Blaney
Senior Olympics
5670 Wilshire Blvd.
Los Angeles, California 90036

The Senior Olympics Program has recently enjoyed exposure on national television, highlighting the manner in which thousands of Americans of all ages have chosen to stay in the game through lifetime competition.

15

Special Precautions

Exercise is the medicine that keeps countless people alive. But like all medicine, it must be taken according to prescription.

KENNETH H. COOPER, M.D.
The New Aerobics

One of the first things we discover when we take an interest in personal fitness is that there are people who will try to talk us out of it. Many of the people involved with the fitness movement have observed that there is a definite backlash. For some reason, sedentary people are often upset by the fact that so many others are doing things that are good for them. These people somehow feel threatened and it makes them angry. Every runner who has been running on the roads for any time at all is familiar with the motorist who seems compelled to harass him, insult him, or even try to force him off the road. There have been several documented cases of runners injured — even killed — by automobiles in which the driver later confessed that he was "trying to scare" the runner or "get him to move off the road."

Such motorists certainly warrant a "special precaution" but I mention them mostly to underscore the fact that you are going to encounter people who don't want you to be fit. Several years ago, when I first got into fitness and lost a considerable amount of weight, all of my slim, fit friends told me I looked great; most of my overweight, unfit friends invariably said something like, "Gee, Ray. You look terrible . . . your face looks drawn." One friend, who happens to be overweight, totally sedentary, and a heavy smoker, described how hoards of joggers passed her home each day — even in cold weather. "That can't be good," she blithely remarked as she exhaled a cloud of smoke. Another sedentary acquaintance insists that large numbers of joggers are dropping dead of heart attacks. If asked the source of his information, he simply shakes his head vaguely and clams up. The point of all this is that the first hazard to your health that you are apt to encounter is the friend or relative who will try to convince you that you should remain just as you are.

Of course there are hazards associated with physical activity. The way one avoids the hazards is through knowledge and common sense — not by avoiding exercise altogether.

When you start your training program, the first thing to consider is the physical examination. In his book *The New Aerobics*, Dr. Kenneth Cooper offers these guidelines for various age groups regarding the physical examination:

Under 30: You can begin exercising if you've had a checkup within the last year and the doctor found nothing wrong with you.

Between 30 and 39: You could have a checkup within three months before you start exercising. The examination should include an electrocardiogram (ECG) taken at rest.

Between 40 and 59: Same as for the 30 to 39 group with one important addition. Your doctor should also take an ECG to check your heart while you are exercising [Stress ECG]. Your pulse rate during this test should approach the level it would during aerobic workout.

Over 59: The same requirements as for the 40 to 59 age group except that the examination should be performed immediately before embarking on any exercise program.

During your physical examination there are certain things that you should discuss with your physician. Even if your doctor doesn't raise all of these issues, it's your responsibility to make sure they are all covered:

1. Does your family have a history of heart disease?
2. Are you a smoker?
3. Have you ever suffered from a chronic illness?
4. Does physical activity cause you to become short of breath?
5. Does simple physical activity (like walking) cause you to experience leg cramps?
6. Do you have any condition that limits your range of motion in any part of your body?

Once you have settled into your exercise and/or sports program, it is important to be able to enjoy your activities without experiencing injury, discomfort, or perhaps, a more serious occurrence. It is no more fun to be benched because of injury than it is to be made sedentary by diseases of disuse. And we don't want to give our sedentary friends the opportunity to say, "Why don't you take it easy and act your age?" So, of course, certain precautions are in order.

Listen to Your Body. The first and foremost precautionary measure you can practice is getting in tune with your body. This book was conceived to assist you to stay in the game throughout your lifetime. It is not a training manual to make you an Olympic gold medal winner. The philosophy of personal growth requires activities geared to personal growth. Feeling good after your workout should be your goal, and listening to your body will help to achieve it. If your activities cause you to feel overly fatigued, ease up a bit. This is especially important when you are engaged in such rigorous activities as running, cycling, swimming, squash, or tennis singles. Older people especially are encouraged to develop a sense of their bodies' limitations and to stay within those limits. Listen to your body . . . don't challenge it!

Be Alert for Danger Signals. Dr. Lenore R. Zohman, a consultant on rehabilitative exercise for the American Heart Association, advises individuals involved in sports or exercise programs — especially older or previously sedentary people — to visit a physician if they should experience any of the following during or after a game or workout:

1. Abnormal heart action: e.g. — pulse becoming irregular; — fluttering, jumping, or palpitations in chest or throat; — sudden bursts of rapid heartbeats; — sudden very slow pulse.

2. Pain or pressure in the center of the chest or the arm or throat precipitated by exercise or following exercise (immediate or delayed).

3. Dizziness, lightheadedness, sudden uncoordination, confusion, cold sweat, glassy stare, pallor, blueness or fainting (immediate).

If your heart rate remains elevated — near your target rate — even 5 to 10 minutes after exercise has been stopped, your exercise was probably too vigorous. Try increasing the intensity of your workout more gradually. Also, keep your pulse rate during your workout on the low end of your target range. If these measures do not bring about a faster recovery to normal heart rate, discuss this problem with your doctor.

Proper Clothing and Footwear. One of the best things to come out of the current enthusiasm for jogging and running is the evolution of truly functional footwear for the active person. Every sporting-goods store in America probably now carries a complete line of "running shoes." If you are going to be jogging or running regularly — even walking — you should have a pair. Here's why: During your jogging or running workout, your feet will strike the ground thousands of times. Your shoe must be light enough so that this doesn't cause strain or fatigue. It must have sufficient cushioning so that it absorbs the repetitive shocks of the foot strike. It should be properly designed so that it doesn't cause painful conditions to occur in the front of the lower leg (shin splints) or in the area below the calf (Achilles' tendinitis). The shoe should have sufficient structural integrity so that it doesn't cause the foot to wobble or pronate as it strikes the ground. All of the top-of-the-line running shoes have all of these qualities. But they are not all identically made. The best way to acquire the right shoes for you is to go to a store specializing in footwear for sports. Tell the sales person how much you run or jog and on what kind of surfaces. He will measure your foot and recommend a shoe. Try it on. If it is the right shoe for you, you will know it. Running shoes are the most comfortable shoes ever designed. Put a pair on and you literally want to run. They are excellent for walking, and many people enjoy wearing them as a casual shoe.

The best type of clothing to wear during exercise sessions or sports activities is very much a matter of common sense. Once you become involved in a sport, for example, you soon learn what kind of clothing is the most functional and comfortable. Cotton apparel seems to be favored for hot weather sports and exercise because of its absorbent qualities. When you first begin to jog, run, or cycle in cold weather, you are likely to overdress. Don't wear heavy bulky clothing; dress in layers — a sweater or two with a light nylon Windbreaker. It is important to be able to remove clothing as you warm up so that you don't sweat too heavily. If you perspire too much and your clothes become sodden, you may end up with a severe chill. Keep your head (and ears) and your hands warm, and you'll be surprised how the rest of your body will adjust to the weather.

Proper Warm-up Before Exercise or Sports. Begin every workout with ten to twenty minutes of warm-up exercises. Use the exercises found in Chapter 10, "Get Loose, Stay Loose." This is important for everyone, but especially for older athletes and exercisers. Warming-up will not only help to prevent muscle pulls and cramps but will eventually become a favorite part of your exercise routine. Once we begin to achieve or restore full range of motion in muscles and joints, we find that the gentle stretching in the warm-up routine truly feels good. And don't forget the cool-down period after your workout.

Children and young adults adjust easily to rigorous exercise. They heal quickly if a muscle is strained or pulled, and they have the resiliency of youth, which enables them to "bounce back" after minor injuries. Those of us in our middle years and older must exercise a bit more cautiously when we work out or play at our sport. That's why it's a good idea to take any unusual aches, pains, or symptoms to our physician. Remember that we decided right in the beginning that our training program was going to be a team effort, with our doctor making up the other half of the team. He'll help keep us off the bench if we give him the chance.

16

The Medical Side

It is not desire that leads to knowledge but necessity.

JOSÉ ORTEGA Y GASSET

By now you know that the orientation of this book is the pursuit of well-being. Almost by definition, a positive approach to aging means the seeking out and implementation of living habits and lifestyles that will result in good general health and the avoidance of illness and disease. When physicians prescribe such an approach to positive health, they call it "preventive medicine." As a "reborn athlete," you are already enjoying the effects of preventive medicine, although, happily, no medicine is involved. "Preventive self-care" might be a better way to describe it. That's not to discount the role of traditional medicine in our lives. The job now is to help your physician help you make preventive medicine a positive force in your life.

One of the ways he can do this is by helping you find one of the preventive medicine facilities in your area. This is a new and exciting dimension of medical practice, and consequently, preventive medicine centers are emerging in many cities throughout the United States. The Strang Clinic in New York is one of the better known. What happens at such centers? They look for disease *before* it occurs by exposing what are called "risk factors." Risk factors take many forms: They can be hereditary, environmental, or tied in with an individual's living habits. We explored this concept earlier in Chapter 2, "Diseases of Choice, Diseases of Disuse." The health professionals at a preventive medicine center often use a team approach — as well as modern technology — to detect possible disease and generation risk factors. As a client at such a center (they often avoid the word patient since you are not sick), you will be given a meticulous physical examination including an exercise stress test and a complete body chemistry work-up. You may be interviewed by a psychologist. You will fill out a lengthy questionnaire concerning your own medical history and that of your family. It will include your eating habits. Finally, all of the information from your physical exam, your interview, and your answers to the questionnaire will be fed into a computer. Out will come your health profile. From this information clinicians will be able to tell you what diseases you have and those you are likely to contract — unless you change your living habits.

Again, based on your personal health profile, the health professional working with you can give you a health plan for positive living and for illness prevention. Such a plan will include modification of lifestyle habits, a nutrition program, and an exercise program — probably much like the one you are using from this book. The value of such a personalized health evaluation is obvious. If you are showing signs that hypertension, heart disease, or some other malady is in the offing, you will have a specific plan to head off the illness and keep you in running order.

In order to give you an idea of how this works, I have included a sample questionnaire used by the preventive medicine practitioners at St. Louis University Medical Center. The questions on the form are designed to predict life expectancy, in years, based on some of the factors mentioned above. Fill it out and check the results. It will give you some idea of where you are right now and how you can stack the cards in your favor.

PHYSICAL FITNESS/POSITIVE LIVING PROGRAM
HOW LONG CAN YOU LIVE?

Want to know how long you can expect to live? Of course, nobody can tell you exactly, but this quiz, based on scientific fact, is more dependable than a crystal ball. (Better still, if you don't like the answer, you can do something about it!)

Here's how to play. First, write down the average expected life span for your sex — 75 for women, 67 for men. (Women and men in their fifties and sixties should add 10 years to this figure because all of you already have proven to be healthy.) Then, as you answer each question below, circle the number of points you score in the Plus or Minus column. Finally, add the total pluses to the average span, subtract the total minuses, and you'll end up with your personal life-expectancy score.

	Plus	*Minus*	*Reason for Score*
Are you a light drinker (2 drinks a day)?	2		A little alcohol aids relaxation; too much is harmful; teetotalers' values may be too rigid.
Are you a heavy drinker (more than 2)?		8	
Are you a teetotaler?		1	
Do you smoke 2 or more packs of cigarettes daily?		8	Studies show chemicals in cigarettes cause lung cancer.
Do you smoke 1 to 2 packs?		4	
Do you smoke less than a pack a day?		2	
Are you a nonsmoker?	2		
Do you exercise moderately (jogging) 3 times weekly?	3		Exercise keeps muscles strong.
Are you happily married?	3		The presence of a "significant other" in one's life is a major plus.
Are you single and between 26 and 35?		1 *	

	Plus	Minus	Reason for Score
Is your job active (house-work, sales work, etc.)?	3		Physical activity is essential for maintaining good muscle tone.
Is your job sedentary (secretarial, other seated work)?		3	
Do you sleep 9 hours a day?		4	Too much sleep saps energy.
Do you sleep 10 or more hours a day?		6	
Have you lived most of your life in an urban environment (e.g., New York)?		1	Urban living creates stress through competition for space, etc. Rural living is more leisurely.
Have you lived most of your life in a rural environment (e.g., the Dakotas)?	1		
Is your family's income over $40,000 per year?		2	Success often brings stress.
Do you have less than a high-school education?		2	Education usually creates increased awareness of proper health care and life planning.
Do you have 4 years of school beyond high school?	1		
Do you have 5 or more years beyond high school?	3		
Are you over 60 and still active?	2		This enhances quality of life.
Is your home's thermostat set at no more than 68°F.?	2		Low temperatures slow body aging.
Are you a reasoned, practical person?	1		Stress caused by aggression and competition shortens life.
Are you aggressive, intense, and competitive?		1	
Are you basically happy and content with life?	1		Stress from unhappiness shortens life.
Are you often unhappy (worried, tense, and guilty)?		1	

	Plus	Minus	Reason for Score
Do you use seat belts regularly, and obey speed limits?	1		Shows a concern for safety.
Are you at least 10 pounds overweight?		1 **	The heart works harder to pump blood through a fat body.
Are you over 40 and not overweight?	3		
If you're a woman over 30, do you give yourself a monthly breast self-examination, have your doctor give you a periodic breast exam and Pap smear?	2		Treatment of cancer is most effective when the disease is caught at an early stage.
If you're a man over 40, do you have an annual medical examination and proctoscopic exam every 2 years?	2		Checkups aid early detection of life-threatening diseases.
Have 2 of your grandparents lived to 80, or beyond?	5		Longevity is hereditary.
Has any parent, grandparent, sister, or brother died of heart attack or stroke before 50?		4	Heredity increases chances of suffering one of these diseases.
Has anyone died from these diseases before 60?		2	
Have there been any cases of diabetes, thyroid disorders, breast cancer, cancer of the digestive system, asthma, emphysema, or chronic bronchitis among parents or grandparents?		3 †	There is a genetic predisposition to these diseases, so odds of getting one are greater — but not inevitable.

TOTALS:

* If you're 36 to 45, it's −2; 46 to 55, −3, etc.   ** For each additional 10 pounds subtract another point.   † Subtract 3 points for each such case. Prepared by Drs. Richard H. Davis and Diana S. Woodruff.

17

Body, Mind, and Soul, The Holistic View

> I took with me certain criteria with which to measure. That which made for more life, for physical and spiritual health was good; that which made for less life, which hurt, dwarfed, and distorted life, was bad.
>
> JACK LONDON
> *People of the Abyss*

A word that is gaining currency in our culture is *holism*. Athletes speak of a "holistic" approach to their sport; modern health professionals are advocating a "holistic" concept of health care and health maintenance. It is an important word because it provides a label for something that many of us have sensed all along: that there is no aspect of mental, spiritual, or physical health or growth that does not involve the entire organism.

An interesting comment on the subject of holism comes from a brochure produced by the Holistic Health Institute in San Diego, California. It reads in part: "The idea of holism and its implications for our human condition has been influential for thousands of years. Holism refers to the theory that whole entities (such as human beings) have an existence and a reality greater than the sum of their parts." The objective, of course, is to apply a holistic philosophy to our daily lives to facilitate our pursuit of health, fitness, and personal growth. The most radical aspect of holism is that it is more than simply caring for all parts of the body. When one part of the body is ailing, it is because, somehow, the holistic harmony of the entity has been disrupted. Such a disruption is likely to have many consequences beyond the pain or infection that commands the greatest attention. Similarly, it can have a wide variety of causes. An aberration of the holistic harmony may be connected to nutrition; perhaps, a vital nutriment has been lacking in the diet. The cause may be due to a lifestyle habit, such as the introduction of toxins into the body through the use of tobacco, drugs, or alcohol. Many people experience illness as a result of stress and tension, especially when they fail to dissipate the effects of tension through exercise or relaxation techniques.

Some readers may find the subject of holism mystical and vague and, perhaps, not as scientific as they would like. It is somewhat mystical because it is not completely understood. But the *scientific* interrelationship of the body, the mind, and the spirit *is* beginning to be understood. Even the medical community has begun to accept the legitimacy of the holistic approach to health care. As more physicians become *wellness* rather than *sickness* oriented, as more of them become involved in *positive* or *preventive* medicine, holistic techniques will become accepted medical procedure. A California pediatric allergist, Dr. Lawrence Podolsky, outlined his views on holistic medicine for his colleagues in *Modern Medicine* magazine (July 15, 1977) in his article, "Wholistic Medicine: What Is It, Who Practices It, Who Needs It?" These are what he calls the principles of the new medicine:

- Disease and sickness engender the greatest medical costs. Prevent them and costs will plummet.
- Anxiety and tension lower a person's resistance. Prophylaxis comes through spiritual awareness and health.
- You are what you eat. Eat wholesomely, and health will follow.
- Symptoms are not synonymous with disease. Allowing an illness to run its course may be better than intervening.

- The most expensive treatment is not necessarily the best.
- The ideal is positive wellness, not just the absence of disease.
- People should be made responsible for their own care and not rely on doctors.
- Drugs and drug reactions cause more harm than good.
- If you haven't tried it (holistic medicine), don't knock it.

Dr. Podolsky's use of the words *spiritual awareness* in his second "principle" above is especially significant. Certainly, it introduces an admittedly unscientific element of the human equation into what has usually been considered an entirely scientific discipline. Although the doctor's last point is addressed to his fellow physicians, it does by implication extend to us, the potential patients. But since we are considering holism as a *wellness* technique, the term *holistic medicine* is inaccurate. By using holism as a tool for positive living, we attempt not only to head off illness but, even more important, to increase our powers to the maximum. This will require a new look at our personal habits and the ways in which they function with each other.

A *Reader's Digest* anthology entitled *Getting the Most Out of Life* was published in 1946, before the holistic approach to life was recognized. The articles in the anthology contained nearly all the elements of holism, but while the editors had recognized that all of the subjects in some way belonged together, each had been presented as a solution to a specific problem. Some of the titles of the articles in the collection included: "Take a Deep Breath" by Helen Durham; "Wake Up and Live" by Dorothea Brande; "It's More Fun to Be Fit" by Gene Tunney; "Making Habits Work for You" by William James; "How to Take a Walk" by Alan Devoe; "Are You a Man or a Smokestack?" by J. P. McEvoy; "How Your Mind May Make You Ill" by Elsie McCormick; "Women Over Forty" by Sarah Trent; "You Can Sleep" by J. P. McEvoy; and "How

to Live on 24 Hours a Day" by Arnold Bennett. All of the subjects were treated separately, in much the same way that
traditional medicine would see them, making little or no con-
nection between a boring (or stressful) job, heavy smoking,
physical lassitude, sexual impotence or disinterest, poor posture, a pot belly, and low back pain. The holistic health specialist might well expect to see all of those characteristics in
a single individual and would regard them as symptoms: symptoms of a damaged, disrupted, faltering, holistic system. The
sad — even frightening — fact is that, in the traditional view,
without the low back pain an individual suffering with all the
other factors would be considered healthy.

As we know now, our spiritual, mental, and physical health
and harmony are primary in determining how kindly the aging
process treats us.

*

In order to utilize the potential of holism to help us establish
our daily growth, achieve health and happiness, and stay in
the game, it is necessary to find a practical approach, to find
an "entry point." "The Self-Care Surge," an editorial in the
October 3, 1977, *Medical World News*, focuses on four in-
gredients that holistic health experts offer as basic to holistic
harmony, which are exercise, proper nutrition, relaxation, and
habit control. But where does one start? With habit control?
We've all had our shot (or shots) at that. With relaxation?
Go tell a tense, uptight person to relax. With nutrition? Perhaps. But most people with poor dietary habits know that they
are not eating properly; they need something to help them
correct that problem. What about exercise? Previous chapters
have outlined the many ways that exercise, physical activity,
and recreational sports help our hearts, lungs, circulatory systems, internal organs, skin, muscles, joints, and the male and
female physique. We have explored how regular, endurance-
type exercise assists us in dissipating tension and nervous en-

ergy; we have seen how such exercise can contribute to our serenity, our confidence, and our ability to concentrate. It would seem that if we engage in a classic strength, flexibility, and endurance exercise program we have this holistic business pretty well licked. Not altogether surprisingly, this is true — at least for many of us.

One of the first clues that this is so came to light as a result of an experiment conducted by the National Aeronautics and Space Administration in the 1960s. Several hundred NASA employees were introduced to a physical fitness program. After a year the results were tabulated and analyzed. Observers were surprised to learn that those who had adhered strictly to the program showed results that transcended mere physical fitness. As opposed to the "nonadherers," the "rigid adherers" showed improved work attitudes and increased job interest and performance, reporting significantly increased ability to deal with the pressures of the job. Smoking, eating, and drinking habits tended to moderate, and nutritious foods began to replace "empty calories." Those who had carefully followed the program also reported an upturn in personal relationships, including sexual interest and activity. Health professionals today would not find these results surprising or unusual.

Exercise is considered now, by most specialists in positive medicine, to be the ideal starting point for changing one's living habits radically. Why? Perhaps it is as simple a matter as *movement*. Movement is life enhancing; the absence of movement is death. The reason that exercise appears to be the most functional entry point into a positive, holistic life cycle hangs on a paradox: Exercise is an independent activity. It is, by itself, totally unconnected with anything else that we do. If one decides to ride a bicycle for an hour a day, it is simply a matter of obtaining a bicycle and finding a convenient hour for cycling. It is a single action. It is not necessary to change anything else about one's living habits to become a cyclist. Thus, the excursion into the new holistic life-plan begins with the decision to adopt an exercise activity. Nothing else is changed; yet, everything else *is* changed, or soon will be. If a well-planned program of regular exercise is undertaken, there is not a cell, not a symptom, not a sense or syndrome that is not affected.

Let's examine that idea and see if it holds water. Think about someone in your life — a friend, relative, or business associate — who has been caught up in the current jogging fever. Not a dilettante but someone who has become a serious runner. Chances are that you have noticed a good many changes in that person, not only in appearance but in lifestyle. For example, the serious runner doesn't smoke. He or she may have known about the hazards of smoking but was unable to stop until becoming a runner. Exercise expert Bob Glover, author of *The Runner's Handbook*, has held jogging clinics for several years for the New York Road Runners. Bob observes that many former smokers have told him that, once they became runners, they automatically cut down on or stopped smoking . . . not so much a volitional thing as a matter of *not needing* that cigarette any longer. Others have made similar observations regarding the intake of food and the use of alcohol. Dr. Emanuel Cheraskin, an Atlanta nutrition specialist, is one of the authors of *Psychodietetics*, a book detailing the relationship between nutrition and emotional health. In the book, Dr. Cheraskin describes experiments involving exercisers and nonexercisers. It seems that when people begin to exercise vigorously and regularly, they also begin to experience subtle changes in their dietary habits. According to Dr. Cheraskin, the exercisers, as opposed to the nonexercisers, instinctively began to choose foods with higher nutritional content, even though their total calorie intake might remain roughly the same. "The exercisers," Dr. Cheraskin says, "had a higher intake of every vitamin, mineral, and amino acid studied. They also consumed far less coffee, tea, alcohol, tobacco, sugar, and refined carbohydrates." Dr. Cheraskin additionally points out that, among the exercising groups, blood-glucose levels are controlled, thus preventing the hypoglycemic cycle with its attendant craving for sweets and stimulants.

The holistic practitioner would see a great deal of sense in Dr. Cheraskin's data, which starkly demonstrate what he understands to be the interaction of lifestyle elements. In Dr. Cheraskin's "exerciser," we have physical activity resulting in an instinctive upgrading of nutrition. This, in turn, produces desirable body-chemistry changes that result in improved health and positive behavior patterns.

One might speculate that, in the holistic view, exercise is a positive, life-enhancing act that stimulates, motivates, and prods one to adopt other life-enhancing activities. It is possible that individual human beings must move in one direction or the other: either embracing a holistic cycle of life-enhancing actions and philosophies or succumbing to a *thanatos* or death-oriented pattern populated with destructive lifestyle habits.

*

If exercise can be the impetus for modifying lifestyles, for replacing destructive habits with positive alternatives, what else can we expect to see happen within the holistic picture? We are, after all, talking about body, mind, and spirit. Since it is impossible to separate these aspects of a person and examine them separately, we will have to step back and observe what other dimensions of daily living are influenced by exercise. The diagram below illustrates the Holistic Health, Self-Care, and Growth Cycle and attempts to show how body, mind, and spirit are influenced by a holistic approach using exercise as the "entry point."

Relaxation, for example, is a mind-body condition essential for emotional stability and for the ability to deal intelligently with life situations. Exercise, of course, is not the only way that we can get our bodies to relax. Transcendental Meditation and other relaxation response techniques are beneficial. They do not have the collateral pluses of exercise, but they are very effective when used in tandem with an exercise program. Out of relaxation, bolstered by the energy generated by exercise, will come a new dimension of productivity.

Another quality that appears to benefit greatly from a regimen of regular exercise is creativity. Consider some of the creative minds possessed by people who exercise. The classical Greeks, for instance, were believers in exercise. Some of the most creative, innovative thinking in Western culture came from Athens, and many of the Greek mathematicians, physicians, and philosophers referred to their "trainers" in their writings. Emerson commented that the extent of his writing was linked to the extent of his walking. " 'Tis one of the secrets for dodging old age," he confided to his friends. Novelist-marathon runner Eric Segal describes a creative stream of consciousness that occurs when he is out on the road; it yields some of his best ideas. "I am often tempted," says Segal, "to dash into a house — right in the middle of a race — ask for a pencil and a piece of paper, and start writing things down." George Sheehan says, "I don't write my columns, I run them."

Several reasons have been suggested for the stimulation of the creative process during exercise, and all of them probably have some validity. First, it should be noted that creative stimulation usually takes place during a rhythmic, endurance-type activity like walking, jogging, cycling, or distance swimming. The rhythmic element suggests a Zen-like consciousness-expansion experience. There is some evidence that the enhanced circulation of oxygen- and nutriment-carrying blood to the brain during exercise helps that organ to function better. Whatever the reason, exercise is central to the phenomenon.

*

Moving to the physical side of the Holistic Cycle diagram, we come to a section labeled "Body Awareness," a term that means very little to the average person but can become quite

Holistic Health, Self-Care, Growth Cycle

Using Exercise as the "Entry Point"

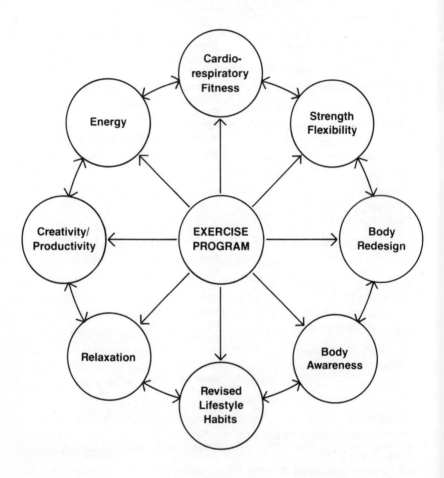

EXERCISE PROGRAM
Jogging, walking, cycling, etc.
Stretching exercises
Strengthening exercises

Cardiorespiratory Fitness
Heart efficiency ↑
Blood pressure ↓
Cardiovascular disease ↓
Pulse rate ↓
Circulation ↑
Cell nourishment and rehabilitation ↑

Energy
Endurance ↑
Fatigue ↓
Work and play capacity ↑
Mental endurance ↑
Initiative ↑
Spiritual and physical vigor ↑

Creativity/Productivity
Confidence ↑
Concentration ↑
Job and hobby interest ↑
Problem solving ↑
Associative and abstract thinking ↑
Spiritual capacity ↑

Relaxation
Sleep ability ↑
Tension ↓
Depression ↓
Mental illness ↓
Interpersonal relationships ↑
Spiritual harmony ↑
Anxiety ↓

Strength Flexibility
Muscular strength ↑
Muscular endurance ↑
Support of internal organs ↑
Posture ↑
Range of body motion ↑
Stiffness ↓
"Aging" of muscles and joints ↓
Sports injuries ↓
Low back pain ↓
Motor skills ↑
Sports abilities ↑

Body Redesign
Fat ↓
Flab ↓
Muscle tone ↑
Muscle mass (men) ↑
Girth ↓
Posture ↑
Figure ↑
Resistance to disease and infection ↑

Body Awareness
Mind-body integration ↑
Sense of limits and capabilities ↑
Likelihood of overdoing stressful
    activities ↓
Personal health "early warning system" ↑

Revised Lifestyle Habits
Overeating ↓
Smoking ↓
Alcohol and drugs ↓
Nutrition ↑
Use of medication ↓

important to those who exercise. Every athlete knows what it means. Olympic gold medal winner Bill Toomey likens the athlete's body to a finely tuned instrument. "You know exactly where you are mentally and physically every instant," says Toomey. "Even in a race, you don't need a stopwatch to tell you how well you're doing . . . you know." Skier Suzy Chaffee tells how a holistic approach to her training enables her to experience a new dimension of her sport. Her body awareness is so complete that she feels as though it extends to her environment. She becomes one with the snow and the mountain. Joggers, runners, cyclists, and swimmers learn this feeling of "oneness" with their bodies and the attendant sensitivity to their physical state. What this can mean to each person is an ability to find new frontiers of joy and experience in the physical life and, perhaps even more important, to develop a personal "early warning system" concerning our health. The first thing that begins to happen to a person who becomes physically fit is that he or she begins to feel better. The body revels in a holistic health environment; it doesn't send out false signals. When something begins to go wrong, you know it.

Finally, a brief word about the spiritual component of the human entity. It would be presumptuous to say much more about it than to acknowledge that we all know it's there. It definitely fits into the holistic scheme of things and it is the one element that each of us must perceive in his or her unique fashion. William James, in *The Varieties of Religious Experience*, saw spirituality in such diverse human experiences as patriotic fervor and dedication to an ideal as well as in religious involvement. We can all feel comfortable with our own version of spirituality as it functions in the holistic cycle.

Exercise, then, is central to staying in the game and if, as George Sheehan likes to point out, our exercise program can also be our play, why . . . the whole shooting match comes free.

Bibliography

Bailey, Covert. *Fit or Fat.* Boston: Houghton Mifflin Company, 1978.

Benson, Herbert, and Miriam Z. Klipper. *The Relaxation Response.* New York: Avon, 1976.

Cheraskin, Emanuel. *Psychodietetics.* New York: Bantam, 1976.

Cooper, Kenneth. *The New Aerobics.* New York: Bantam, 1970.

Cureton, Thomas K. *The Physiological Effects of Exercise Programs on Adults.* Springfield, Illinois: Charles C Thomas, 1969.

Fixx, James P. *The Complete Book of Running.* New York: Random House, 1977.

Higdon, Hal. *Fitness After Forty.* Mountain View, California: World Publications, 1977.

Huizinga, Johan. *Homo Ludens: A Study of the Play-Element in Culture.* Boston: Beacon Press, 1955.

Glover, Bob, and Jack Shepherd. *The Runner's Handbook: A Complete Fitness Guide for Men and Women on the Run.* New York: Penguin, 1978.

Kostrubala, Thaddeus. *The Joy of Running.* Philadelphia and New York: Lippincott, 1976.

Kraus, Hans. *Backache, Stress and Tension.* New York: Pocket Books, 1969.

Kugler, Hans J. *Slowing Down the Aging Process.* Moonachie, New Jersey: Pyramid Publications, 1973.

Lance, Kathryn. *Running for Health and Beauty.* New York: Bobbs-Merrill, 1977.

Leonard, George. *The Ultimate Athlete.* New York: Avon, 1974.

May, Rollo. *The Courage to Create.* New York: W. W. Norton, 1975.

Pelletier, Kenneth R. *Mind as Healer, Mind as Slayer.* New York: Delta, 1977.

Pritikin, Nathan, with Patrick McGrady, Jr. *The Pritikin Program for Diet and Exercise.* New York: Grosset and Dunlap, 1979.

Selye, Hans. *The Stress of Life.* New York: McGraw-Hill, 1978.

Sheehan, George. *Running and Being.* New York: Simon and Schuster, 1978.

Sheldon, William H. *Atlas of Men.* New York: Hafner, 1970.

Siegener, Ray. *Shape Up for Sports.* New York: Berkley Publications, 1978.

Sussman, Aaron, and Ruth Goode. *Walking.* New York: Fireside, 1967.

Zohman, Lenore. *Exercise Your Way to Health and Fitness.* New York: American Heart Association, 1974.